PARKINSON'S DISEASE
FOR THE HOSPITALIST

Parkinson's Disease *for* *the* Hospitalist

MANAGING THE COMPLEX CARE
OF A VULNERABLE POPULATION

Hooman Azmi, MD FAANS
& Fiona Gupta, MD

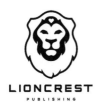

LIONCREST
PUBLISHING

PARKINSON'S DISEASE FOR THE HOSPITALIST

Managing the Complex Care of a Vulnerable Population

ISBN   978-1-5445-1189-4 *Paperback*

      978-1-5445-1190-0 *Ebook*

This book is dedicated to our patients and their caretakers.

They teach and inspire us each and every day.

Contents

Acknowledgments

I would like to acknowledge the Parkinson's DSC team at Hackensack University Medical Center, who have taken ownership of the care of Parkinson's patients in the hospital; the nursing staff; physical and occupational and speech therapy staff; pharmacy staff; and all throughout the hospital who have given so much time and are becoming part of the solution.

In particular, a special thank you to Lisa Coccoziello, Renee Harvee, Nilesh Desai, Peggy McGee, Anthony Rocco, Karen Keeting, Jewell Thomas, Blessy Jacob, Claire Gibbons, Christopher Gazdick, Donna Cricco, Cathy Theiss, Cathryn Monaghan, Eugenia Ndiaye, Christopher Garcia, Lia Kondos, Bridget Wertz, Deena Peretti, Matthew Reigle, and Drs. Patrick Roth, Andy Hummel, and Florian Thomas.

Finally, I would like to thank my colleagues at North Jersey Brain & Spine Center for their endless support and vision.

—HOOMAN AZMI, MD FAANS

Introduction

Time after time, as physicians specializing in the care of people with Parkinson's disease (PD), we have seen our patients receive poor care during hospitalization. When healthcare providers are unfamiliar with the special needs of PD patients, particularly their need for timely administration of medication, patients' conditions can spiral out of control. A patient with PD may end up in worse condition than on admission.

People come to the hospital for many reasons. Sometimes the reason is elective, such as a scheduled surgery for a rotator cuff tear, or the reason is more urgent, such as an active myocardial infarction. Patients with PD are no different. Their admission to the hospital can be elective or urgent, and the majority of these admissions are unrelated to PD. Yet the hospital stay can cause a cascade of unnecessary complications and poor outcomes for patients with PD. A patient's condition can worsen rapidly when hospital staff are unprepared for the care of PD patients. An independent patient who would otherwise be discharged to home may end up needing rehabilitation or nursing home care as the result of poor attention to their PD.

Our goal with this book is to provide a clear, basic understanding of PD, its treatment, and the optimal care of patients during hospitalization. Our recommendations are based on years of experience treating these patients in both the clinic and hospital settings, as well as recommendations from national advocacy groups. We've created this guide as a way to help anyone who happens to come across a patient who has PD, whether in a hospital, a rehabilitation facility, or nursing home, to learn how to avoid complications and *achieve better outcomes.*

USING THIS BOOK

We begin with Part I: Understanding Parkinson's Disease. In this part, we discuss the epidemiology and pathophysiology of the disease, explain how it is diagnosed, and discuss how it is classified and staged.

From there, we go on to Part II: Treatment. We explain the pharmacological and surgical treatments, including a detailed discussion of drug treatments. We proceed to describe the symptoms in detail and the importance of a good multidisciplinary team for helping patients stay safe from complications while admitted to the hospital and maintain an active and independent life.

In Part III: Admission: Problems and Solutions, we discuss the serious issue of incomplete assessment, stress the importance of medication timing, and explore other concerns of the admitted Parkinson's patient. This part deals more specifically with issues around hospitalizations and discusses the experience of two not-so-hypothetical patients.

BETTER OUTCOMES

Parkinson's disease can be challenging to diagnose and treat. Every patient presents differently, progresses differently, and requires an individualized and often complex treatment regimen. All PD patients, however, face similar issues during hospitalization. Careful attention to potential problems, such as mismanagement of medications and administration of contraindicated medications, will help keep hospital stays for PD patients as brief and safe as possible. Most importantly for good outcomes, all Parkinson's patients must always get their medications on time.

When healthcare providers have a solid understanding

of the issues around Parkinson's disease, they're better equipped to treat these patients. The more informed they are, the better able they are to deliver good care, keeping patients safe and family members more satisfied by the care, with fewer complications and a shorter length of stay.

PART I

UNDERSTANDING PARKINSON'S DISEASE

CHAPTER 1

Epidemiology and Pathophysiology

Parkinson's disease was first described by an English physician, Dr. James Parkinson, just over 200 years ago. In 1817, Dr. Parkinson published "Essay on the Shaking Palsy," in which he documented the common symptoms of what he called paralysis agitans. His observations were based on his own patients and also observation on some people he saw on the streets of London. It wasn't until a century later that the great French neurologist Jean-Martin Charcot named the disease in honor of Dr. Parkinson.

Today, we still diagnose PD much as Dr. Parkinson himself did—with a thorough history and clinical exam. We know much more than he did about the disease, and we have many more tools to treat it, but the diagnosis is still made the same way. No blood test or scan can accurately diagnose PD. Physicians can base their diagnoses only on a careful history and the signs and symptoms revealed by the clinical exam.

Parkinson's disease is a chronic, progressive neurodegenerative disease in which voluntary movement becomes more and more impaired over time. PD affects voluntary movement and causes stiffness and spasticity, but patients also have a range of nonmotor symptoms, such as sleep issues, constipation, pain, paresthesias, hallucinations, and cognitive impairment.

After Alzheimer's disease, PD is the most common neurodegenerative disease in America. About five million Americans have Alzheimer's disease; one million Americans have been diagnosed with PD. Because we now have earlier diagnosis and better treatments, people with PD are living longer, healthier lives.

About 60,000 new cases of PD are diagnosed each year. The number of new patients is expected to double by 2030 and triple by 2050. The chief risk factor for developing Parkinson's disease is simply getting older. Most people are diagnosed in their sixties or older, so as the population ages, the number of PD cases will rise.

THE PATHOPHYSIOLOGY OF PD

Parkinson's disease is a manifestation of dopaminergic neuron depletion over time. Dopamine is a neurotransmitter in the brain. Dopamine is produced in the dopaminergic neurons in the ventral tegmental area (VTA) of the midbrain, the substantia nigra pars compacta, and the arcuate nucleus of the hypothalamus.

By the time the diagnosis of Parkinson's is finally made, most patients have already lost about 50 to 70 percent of the dopaminergic neurons of the substantia nigra, which is part of a group of nuclei responsible for relaying and refining multiple circuits in the brain, called the basal ganglia. The prodromal stage for PD is lengthy, with nonspecific symptoms such as constipation, depression, and sleep disorders appearing long before motor symptoms arise. The early symptoms of PD are often vague and easily attributed to other causes, however, and PD is not usually diagnosed until motor symptoms become apparent.

The significant neuronal loss of substantia nigra leads to depletion of dopamine production. Recent thinking about PD by Dr. Heiko Braak suggests that Lewy bodies (misfolded clumps or aggregates inside a nerve cell of a protein called alpha-synuclein) may be behind the death of the dopaminergic cells. This hypothesis suggests PD may actually be caused by misfolding of proteins or errors in the cellular "cleanup" mechanism to break down these proteins, similar to the tangled tau proteins seen in Alzheimer's disease. In PD, the accumulation of Lewy bodies within the neuron damages them, depleting the amount of dopamine that is produced. As this neurotransmitter is depleted, the basal ganglia circuitry, which facilitates normal movement, is disrupted.

Other neurotransmitters are also implicated in Parkinson's disease. In the pathway of progression proposed by Dr. Braak and his team of neuropathologists, PD begins in the medulla oblongata, where norepinephrine is made. Alpha-synuclein deposition then progressively increases. As the disease progresses, the substantia nigra is affected and dopamine loss occurs. From there, as the cortex gets involved, depletion of acetylcholine and other neurotransmitters occurs.

The progressive depletion of all the neurotransmitters is likely why PD has so many different symptoms. When serotonin is depleted, for example, people with PD develop anxiety, depression, and sleep issues. The lack of norepinephrine accounts for a nonmotor symptom called rapid eye movement behavior disorder (REMBD); the lack of acetylcholine affects cognition.

Previous researchers believed PD originates in the substantia nigra. The Braak hypothesis suggests the disease begins long before it reaches the substantia nigra. This alternative explanation is supported by the chronological appearance of autonomic, motor, and cognitive symptoms as the disease progresses. The Braak hypothesis opens the way for research into earlier detection and possible biomarkers by looking at nonmotor symptoms and alpha-synuclein levels.

WHY PEOPLE GET PD

We're not exactly sure why people get Parkinson's disease. The "two-hit" theory suggests the disease is probably caused by a combination of genetic and environmental factors. When an individual who is already genetically predisposed to Parkinson's is then exposed to something from the environment, the combination starts the cascade that culminates in neurotransmitter loss.

We still don't know exactly what in the environment triggers PD or how long the exposure needs to be. Pesticides, herbicides, well water, and rural living have all been hypothesized as causes, but solid evidence is lacking.

Some forms of PD have genetic aspects. So far, about 20 to 30 genes related to PD have been mapped, but the research on this is preliminary. True genetic Parkinson's is rare, however. Most people with Parkinson's have no family history of the disease.

Simply getting older is the largest risk factor for PD. The average patient is diagnosed in their sixties or seventies, but the age range is varied. We see PD quite often in patients younger than 50 and even sometimes younger than 40. Young-onset Parkinson's disease (YOPD) is a genetic form that usually occurs in people younger than 40.

DIAGNOSING PD

Parkinson's disease is difficult to diagnose and can be challenging to treat. Patients often don't present in a typical fashion. As there's still no reliable blood test or scan for PD, diagnosis continues to depend on a good history and a good clinical exam. Often, patients have comorbidities or confounding factors or an unclear history; it is not common to make the diagnosis on a first visit.

We often need to follow up with consecutive visits or try a medication challenge and see how the patient responds. We need to apply clinical judgment to objective and subjective findings and make an accurate diagnosis.

Certain symptoms occur in most PD patients. Known as cardinal features, they aid in making the diagnosis. Cardinal features include:

- Bradykinesia (slowed movement)

- Resting tremor
- Limb rigidity
- Postural instability

To be diagnosed with PD, the person must have bradykinesia and at least one other cardinal feature.

Resting tremor is a high-frequency tremor, with low to moderate amplitude, that occurs when the limb is supported against gravity—when it's at rest. Resting tremor is commonly seen when the person's arm and hand rest on their lap and shake. If the patient is distracted, the tremor might get stronger, but if the patient focuses on the tremor, sometimes they're able to suppress it.

While cardinal features help with the diagnosis of PD, what is challenging about the disorder is how different each patient can be in terms of overall symptoms, response to treatment, and progress of the disease.

PD AND PARKINSON-LIKE SYNDROMES

Idiopathic Parkinson's disease is the most common type of disorder in this category and what we often mean by the term *typical Parkinson's disease*. Parkinson-like syndromes, also called Parkinson-plus syndromes, or atypical Parkinson's, can easily be confused with true PD. These syndromes include:

- Progressive supranuclear palsy (PSP)
- Multisystem atrophy (MSA)
- Corticobasal ganglionic degeneration (CBGD)
- Lewy body dementia
- Drug-induced Parkinsonism
- Vascular Parkinsonism

All these syndromes are characterized by slow, stiff movement and trouble signaling from the brain to the body, but the progress and pathophysiology for each are very different and they each have a different pattern of symptoms. In Lewy body dementia, for example, patients have cognitive symptoms early on, including profound hallucinations, psychosis, and dementia. Vascular Parkinsonism is caused by multiple strokes or ministrokes that affect the white matter of the brain and can cause difficulty with gait (gait apraxia).

Two factors in general distinguish PD and Parkinson-plus syndromes. The time frame of disease advancement varies between these two categories. The rate of progression is usually significantly more accelerated for the atypical forms. Another distinguishing factor is the response to drug treatment. People with typical or idiopathic PD usually respond well to levodopa therapy, while people with the atypical forms respond only minimally or not at all.

As mentioned previously, because PD can vary so much from person to person, diagnosis can be challenging. It is important to seek the expertise of a movement disorders specialist to be able to arrive at the correct diagnosis and appropriate treatment.

PD EPIDEMIOLOGY AND PATHOPHYSIOLOGY

EPIDEMIOLOGY	PD is a chronic progressive neurodegenerative disease
	Voluntary movement becomes increasingly impaired over time
	1+ million people living with PD
	60,000 new patients annually
	Most patients are aged 60+
	Burden of PD expected to double by 2030
PATHOPHYSIOLOGY	Characterized by loss of dopamine
	Lewy bodies damage dopaminergic cells of substantia nigra
	Loss of other neurotransmitters
	Etiology usually unknown
	Most cases are spontaneous
	Age is the largest risk factor

CHAPTER 2

Diagnosis

As mentioned previously, Parkinson's disease is diagnosed by its signs and symptoms, based on a thorough history and physical examination. Here, we discuss the clinical findings that suggest PD and ultimately lead to the diagnosis.

HOW IS THE DIAGNOSIS MADE?

Previously, we discussed the cardinal features of Parkinson's disease. While each patient with PD may have a unique constellation and degrees of symptoms, these cardinal features are what we know to be generally common to patients with PD and help us in making the diagnosis. They are bradykinesia, resting tremor, limb rigidity, and postural instability. Bradykinesia is the presence of slowness of movement, often with an impaired ability to adjust the body's position.

For a diagnosis of PD, bradykinesia must be accompanied by at least one other cardinal feature:

- Resting tremor
- Limb rigidity
- Postural instability

TREMOR

Resting tremor is commonly seen when the patient's arm and hand shake while resting on their lap. Sometimes this is called a "pill rolling" tremor because of how the thumb and index finger move against each other.

Tremor is another very common sign, but a patient can have Parkinson's without a tremor, or with a tremor that is very mild or unnoticeable. The absence of tremor should not be mistaken for the absence of PD.

Conversely, tremor alone does not necessarily mean Parkinson's disease. Essential tremor, the most common movement disorder, causes unintentional trembling or shaking movements in one or more parts of the body. Essential tremor most commonly affects the hands but can also occur in the arms, head, face, vocal cords, trunk, and legs. People with essential tremor are usually over age 40 and are otherwise healthy. Essential tremor may worsen over time, but it doesn't lead to other symptoms or PD.

LIMB RIGIDITY

Limb rigidity is stiffness or "tightness" in the arms and legs and often also the trunk; the limb shows increased resistance when stretched, beyond the resistance that would be expected in an older adult. Cogwheel rigidity is defined as muscular rigidity that causes a stop-and-start movement, like a ratchet, when a limb is moved passively through its range of motion. Although almost all people with PD develop some level of limb rigidity, not all have cogwheel rigidity. Limb rigidity is usually asymmetric and doesn't affect every limb.

POSTURAL INSTABILITY

Postural instability can take many forms. For most people, it's a gait imbalance that causes a shuffling gait. Many people show diminished arm swing when walking. Retropulsion, or spontaneous backward falls, can occur in later stages of Parkinson's. Gait freezing occurs when a patient freezes mid-stride while walking or has start hesitation, where they stand up but can't move any further. Gait freezing in particular can lead to falls. The freezing usually lasts for only a few seconds, but it's hard to overcome. Postural instability gets worse as the disease progresses, and many people end up relying on canes or walkers. Postural instability can cause people to have a stooped or forward-flexed posture while walking, standing, and even sitting.

Two out of four motor symptoms mean PD is clinically possible; three out of four motor symptoms means it's clinically probable.

OTHER MOTOR SYMPTOMS

Parkinson's disease is a head-to-toe disorder that has a range of other motor symptoms:

- Speech hypophonia, or speech that is very soft or low volume, is a common symptom. Other speech difficulties include trouble finding words, stuttering, and speaking in a monotone.
- Dysphagia, or swallowing problems. Dysphagia can range from minor swallowing difficulties to profound, to the point of needing a feeding tube.
- Esophageal dysmotility, or slow passage to the esophagus.
- Facial hypomimia, or a lack of motor facial expression (often described as "masked" expression). This can be seen as diminished eye blinking or a statuesque, unmoving face. The face shows little or no animation when the patient laughs, for example.
- Dystonia, or involuntary muscle contractions resulting in twisting and repetitive movements. The contractions are sometimes painful.
- Gastroparesis, or poor emptying of stomach contents. This causes delayed absorption of medication and food nutrients.

- Dyskinesia, or abnormal, uncontrolled involuntary movements. In people with PD, dyskinesia is usually seen as writhing movements that are caused by long-term use of levodopa therapy, particularly at higher dosages. (We'll discuss this further in chapter 4.)

NONMOTOR SYMPTOMS

Think of PD as an iceberg. Compared to what you can see on the surface, much more is under the water. By the time a diagnosis of PD is made, much more is going on with the patient than the visible motor symptoms. Many brain areas are involved.

Nonmotor symptoms develop along with the motor symptoms and can get worse as the disease progresses. Apathy, anxiety, dementia, autonomic issues, urinary issues, constipation, and other nonmotor symptoms often become more disabling than the visible motor symptoms.

Nonmotor symptoms aren't caused only by dopamine depletion in the brain. As discussed previously, other neurotransmitters, including serotonin, norepinephrine, and acetylcholine, are also low. As the disease continues, the lack of neurotransmitters causes, and compounds, the nonmotor symptoms. In PD, the pathology affects areas in which these neurotransmitters are produced. Premotor symptoms are thought to be because of the involvement of the raphe nuclei and the locus coeruleus in the brain stem. These areas are where norepinephrine and serotonin are made.

NEUROPSYCHIATRIC ISSUES

People with Parkinson's can develop neuropsychiatric issues as the disease progresses, but sometimes these issues precede motor symptoms. The most common problems affecting mood and behavior in PD include:

- Apathy, or lack of emotion, social withdrawal, and general lack of interest
- Anxiety, or excessive uneasiness, worry, and apprehension
- Impulsivity, or behavior with little or no forethought or concern for the consequences
- Depression, or persistent feelings of sadness or hopelessness, loss of interest in favorite activities, excessive tiredness, thoughts of death or suicide, and other symptoms
- Psychosis, or disruptions of thought and perception that cause some loss of contact with reality. Patients with PD may experience psychosis that includes hallucinations and paranoia
- Cognitive impairment, which can range from mild all the way up to full-blown dementia

APATHY

Apathy is sometimes difficult to distinguish from depression. Apathy is basically lack of motivation. Activities that used to be pleasurable, such as going out to lunch or seeing friends, stop being of interest. People with PD who are depressed are often also apathetic, but they will have additional symptoms that will distinguish apathy from depression.

BRADYPHRENIA

The most common cognitive issue in Parkinson's is bradyphrenia, or slowness of thinking. PD patients commonly develop difficulty with cognitive processing but not because they have dementia or even mild cognitive impairment. Instead, the processing speed in their brain has slowed down. For example, if a PD patient goes out to dinner with several other people, they may have trouble keeping up with the conversation. Bradyphrenia also causes difficulty with word finding.

Caregivers and healthcare providers should be aware of bradyphrenia in PD patients. When discussing the plan of care, for example, you may need to repeat your points and go slowly to be sure the patient is following you and processing the information. Bradyphrenia isn't a problem with comprehension; it's a delay in processing, like having a time lag.

DEMENTIA

Dementia is usually a later symptom in Parkinson's. As the disease progresses, more of the brain becomes involved. The disorder affects the lower brainstem and then moves up to the substantia nigra, which is in the midbrain. When it reaches that point, Parkinson's symptoms start. The disease continues to progress up into the mesocortex and the neocortex. The neocortex is responsible for higher-order brain functions, such as cognition, vision, spatial reasoning, and language. Because the disorder usually reaches this area years after PD has started, dementia usually happens late in the disease progression. The Sydney Multicenter Study found that at around 12 to 15 years after diagnosis, about 70 percent of patients had some degree of dementia. At 20 years, the percentage rose to 90. The longer someone has Parkinson's, the higher the chance of developing dementia.

In the later stages of PD, dementia may include short- and long-term memory impairment, issues with judgment, impulsivity, and diminished cognitive processing.

Dementia is a prominent nonmotor symptom, and the incidence increases as the disease advances. Caregivers and healthcare providers should always take the possibility of dementia into consideration when working with a patient with Parkinson's.

PSYCHOSIS

Some reports suggest that up to 50 percent of patients with PD may have psychosis at some point. The psychosis may be caused by the neuropathology of the disease, or it may be caused by external factors, such as the medications the patient is taking, or both.

Psychosis usually manifests with more positive symptoms, as opposed to disorders such as schizophrenia, which generally have more negative symptoms. For people with PD, the most common symptom of psychosis are visual hallucinations. Less frequently, patients can also have auditory hallucinations. Even less common are tactile hallucinations, causing them to constantly feel as if something is crawling on them or to feel an itchy sensation. Olfactory hallucinations that affect the sense of smell can also occur.

When helping a patient with psychosis, it is key to notice whether the patient has insight or not while the hallucination is happening or afterward. Most PD patients typically will have insight and be aware that their hallucinations aren't real. They'll say, "I saw my mother sitting at the table with me, but I know she's not really there." Even when a patient has insight into their hallucinations, however, they're still upsetting to experience.

When insight into hallucinations becomes lost, treatment

becomes much more difficult. PD patients can start to develop delusions, including paranoia and often persecutory delusions. Development of difficult-to-treat psychosis can make the care of the patient in the home even more difficult and can lead to long-term facility placement. For patients who have psychosis, the mortality rate can be as high as 30 percent in three years.

DELIRIUM

Delirium is extremely common among hospitalized Parkinson's patients. It's important to establish a diagnosis of Parkinson's psychosis prior to hospitalization if possible. During the hospital stay, keeping an eye on the patient's mental status is crucial. Changes should be noted. It is important to note that one of the most common causes of delirium in a PD patient admitted to the hospital is delay in administration of PD medications or administration of contraindicated medications. (We'll discuss this in detail later in the book.)

SLEEP-RELATED SYMPTOMS

Most people with PD have sleep disorders that often predate diagnosis. Rapid eye movement behavior disorder (REMBD) is a common problem. In this condition, patients may cry out in their sleep, act out their dreams, have vivid dreams (parasomnia), and thrash out while sleeping.

In addition to REMBD, sleep fragmentation is a common symptom of PD. People with PD can usually fall asleep normally but will wake up every few hours. They don't get a consistent level of sleep. Restless leg syndrome is also a problem for PD patients and can cause significant sleep loss. Another common problem is nocturia, where a patient needs to get up to urinate every few hours, further disrupting sleep. Nocturia in PD patients is a significant problem that should be treated with appropriate medication. Difficulties with sleep in PD patients can lead to daytime sleepiness and sometimes an overwhelming need to sleep (sleep attacks).

PD inpatients with sleep disorders find that the noisy hospital environment often affects their sleep negatively. They often just don't sleep at all at night. Their daytime symptoms get worse, so they're then given sleep medications. That can cause a vicious circle of worsening problems, because many PD patients will respond paradoxically to the drugs and be more wakeful at night and even sleepier during the day.

As we get older in general, our sleep quality declines. Many people with PD are in their seventies, eighties, and even older and have the usual sleep quality issues associated with their age along with PD sleep disorders. For Parkinson's patients, it's really important to be aware of sleep issues and advocate for the best sleep patterns possible for them. This is especially key for inpatients. In our experience, sleep problems such as REMBD that occur in the hospital often aren't recognized as intrinsic to the disease and are seen as having a different cause. Some patients end up coming out of the hospital on antipsychotic drugs because the clinician didn't realize they had a PD-related sleep disorder, not nighttime hallucinations.

Treatment of sleep-related disorders is paramount in treating Parkinson's disease, especially for hospitalized patients. Selecting the right agent for treatment is key. (The best sleeping medications for PD patients will be discussed in chapter 4.)

Sleep hygiene is also critical. Ideally, the patient will go to bed at the same time every night, with minimal disruptions, no TV, and a cool, dark room. It would be ideal if that could actually be done in a hospital or rehab setting.

AUTONOMIC SYMPTOMS

The autonomic nervous system is entirely different from the motor and nonmotor systems. The autonomic nervous system controls basic bodily functions such as respiration. Over time, people with PD will almost always develop autonomic system problems.

Blood pressure is maintained and regulated by the autonomic nervous system. When we move from lying or sitting to standing, baroreceptors in the heart sense pressure changes and trigger a baroreflex response by the autonomic nervous system. The hormone norepinephrine, which helps to maintain blood pressure, is released and peripheral vasoconstriction is activated, all to maintain a constant cerebral blood flow. The baroreceptor response ensures that our blood pressure, and therefore cerebral blood flow, stays the same when we move from sitting to standing.

People with PD lose this baroreceptor response, especially as the disease advances. When the baroreceptor response doesn't activate immediately, the patient may experience orthostatic (postural) hypotension: the blood pressure goes from normal to high normal and drops noticeably when the patient stands up. The drop is defined as either 20 mm mercury systolic, or 10 mm diastolic, within three minutes of standing up. The drop probably happens because they don't release norepinephrine and peripheral vasoconstriction is hampered, although we're still not sure about this.

Because they lack an effective baroreceptor response, patients can get lightheaded, dizzy, or nauseous; space out; or freeze when they move from lying or sitting to standing. The result is that a PD patient is at risk of falling every time they stand up.

In the inpatient setting, it is extremely important to be aware of the fall risk for any PD patient. When helping a patient out of bed, do it slowly. Recline the bed up, or have them sit on the edge of the bed and then stand up slowly. Have them stand up slowly from a seated position. Stay close and be alert to the fall risk.

When taking the blood pressure of a Parkinson's patient, measure not only the seated or reclining blood pressure but also the orthostatic blood pressure. If orthostatic hypotension is detected, awareness will help prevent falls.

Orthostatic hypotension can be helped with nondrug treatments. Make sure PD patients don't lie flat, especially when sleeping. This can lead to supine hypertension, where the blood pressure rises when the patient is flat. When the patient also has orthostatic hypotension, the drop in blood pressure when they get up is even greater and more likely to cause dizziness and falls when going from flat to sitting or standing. Supine hypertension can be avoided by elevating the head of the bed by at least 60 degrees. This is easily done in a hospital bed. In a standard bed, a wedge pillow can be used.

Hydration is crucial. When patients are dehydrated, they

tend to be more prone to orthostasis. Adequate salt intake is also key. PD patients can develop postprandial hypotension in which blood pressure falls by 20 mm systolic 15 to 90 minutes after a meal. Postprandial hypotension happens most often in the morning, so eating something salty at breakfast, such as salted peanuts or pretzels, can help maintain the blood pressure. Compression stockings can also be helpful. These typically have to be up to the abdomen to be effective.

If nonpharmacological measures don't help or don't help enough, drugs can be used. Fludrocortisone (Florinef), a peripheral mineral corticoid, can be effective. It's a tablet that's very easy to administer and is usually needed only once a day in the morning. Plasma expanders, such as midodrine (Amatine, ProAmatine), expand intravascular volume and raise blood pressure. This drug usually has to be given three times a day. The only approved drug is droxidopa (Northera), which works centrally as a norepinephrine precursor.

Urinary Incontinence

Urinary symptoms in PD are quite profound and prominent. Patients can have:

- Urinary frequency in which they frequently have to use the bathroom

- Urinary urgency in which they get the urge to use the bathroom but might not fully empty the bladder
- Frank incontinence in which they are unable to void
- Nocturia, or frequent urination at night

The urinary issues of PD mean these patients are also very prone to urinary tract infections. Urinary incontinence is distressing to patients. Having a urologist on the treatment team who is really on board with these patients and familiar with the urological manifestations of PD can be very helpful.

Gastrointestinal Issues

Parkinson's is a head-to-toe disorder, and gastrointestinal (GI) issues affect many patients. Constipation is extremely common for PD patients, but dysfunction often extends to the entire GI tract.

Excessive saliva, drooling, and swallowing issues are common. Esophageal dysmotility can also occur. The patient gets esophageal reflux or has dysmotility issues throughout the esophagus.

Gastroparesis, or slow stomach motility, is another common problem. It's important to be aware of gastroparesis because it affects how medication is absorbed. When a patient takes levodopa, the effects usually are seen in 15 or 20 minutes. When a patient has gastroparesis, however, the effect can take an hour, as the pill sits in the stomach.

Constipation is a common premotor symptom and often predates the diagnosis of PD. Constipation in Parkinson's is defined as the inability to go for three days. It can be very disabling and is a common cause of emergency room visits and hospitalizations. As with other nonmotor symptoms, we encourage nonpharmacological treatments, such as adequate hydration and exercise. For drug treatment, we don't really have a preferred go-to product. Many patients use nonprescription laxatives or MiraLAX (polyethylene glycol); some use suppositories.

The range of gut issues experienced by PD patients is a good argument for including a GI specialist on the treatment team.

Medication mismanagement can compound GI symptoms while the patient is admitted to the hospital, causing dysphagia and GI dysfunction. When a patient is admitted, it is crucial to adhere to their home medication regime to help reduce or prevent these issues.

PREMOTOR SYMPTOMS

Premotor symptoms often predate the onset of the cardinal symptoms of Parkinson's. A very early symptom that can predate the diagnosis of Parkinson's is handwriting changes. Micrographia, or abnormally small handwriting, is common. Patients also find it difficult to draw a spiral.

Another early premotor symptom is the loss of smell (anosmia), which eventually affects almost all PD patients. This is probably because the olfactory bulb is involved very early on, before other symptoms appear. Sleep disorders are very common and are a huge premotor predictor of Parkinson's. Other early signs of PD include anxiety and depression.

Premotor symptoms of PD can start five years or more before more obvious and specific motor symptoms begin. Some data show that premotor symptoms can predate Parkinson's by 10 or maybe even 20 years. Any one premotor symptom isn't sufficient to suspect PD. Depression might just be depression; constipation might just be constipation. The conglomeration of symptoms, however, should heighten clinical suspicion.

PD SYMPTOMS

MOTOR SYMPTOMS	NONMOTOR SYMPTOMS	PREMOTOR SYMPTOMS
Tremor at rest	Depression and apathy	Olfactory dysfunction (anosmia)
Rigidity	Bradyphrenia	Depression and anxiety
Bradykinesia	Psychosis	Rapid eye movement behavior disorder (REMBD)
Postural/gait disturbances	Sleep disorders including REMBD	Constipation
Stooped or forward-flexed posture	Blood pressure fluctuations	
Handwriting changes	Urinary incontinence	
	Constipation	

CHAPTER 3

Staging and Rating of Parkinson's Disease

Different scales and scoring systems are used for staging Parkinson's disease. They all aim to convey the state of advancement in PD in a patient. Familiarity with these scales is important, as they give healthcare providers a sense of how affected and how medication-dependent a patient may be.

STAGING PD

Two main scales are used to stage PD: the Hoehn and Yahr scale and the Movement Disorder Society Unified Parkinson's Disease Rating Scale™ (MDS-UPDRS). When a patient enters the hospital, it isn't realistic or necessary for the admitting nurse or doctor to score and stage the patient. Familiarity with the score, however, is useful. It's a good reference point that helps the staff know what to expect from a PD patient.

While there are five stages of PD, patients can vary considerably within their staging. In addition, some will progress rapidly through the stages, and others will progress more slowly or reach a particular stage and not progress further. We have no way of determining when a patient might reach a particular stage or how long they might remain there.

HOEHN AND YAHR SCALE

The Hoehn and Yahr scale uses an established 1 through 5 staging system based on motor symptoms:

- Stage 1. Symptoms are very mild; only one side of the body affected (unilateral involvement). In general, these patients aren't terribly affected by their PD.
- Stage 2. Both sides of the body affected (bilateral involvement), but balance isn't impaired. This stage is also considered early PD. Dependence on medication isn't as pronounced as in the later stages.
- Stage 3. Mild to moderate bilateral disease; some postural instability with balance problems, gait disturbances, retropulsion, and increased risk of falls; still

physically independent. These patients are beginning to be affected by their PD symptoms and are highly dependent on their medications.

- Stage 4. Severe disability; cane, walker, or wheelchair may be needed; patient needs help with activities of daily living.
- Stage 5. Very debilitated; wheelchair-bound or bedridden.

UPDRS

The Hoehn and Yahr scale is a good way to describe how the symptoms of Parkinson's progress, but it doesn't consider other aspects of the disease. A more comprehensive rating scale, the UPDRS (Unified Parkinson's Disease Rating Scale), was developed to take many different aspects into account, including cognitive status, subjective status, activities of daily living, and objective medical examination. It also assesses motor fluctuations—the symptoms that occur when the patient is in the "on" state (medication is working) or in the "off" state (medication has worn off or isn't working). The UPDRS rates four areas:

- Part I. Mentation, behavior, mood. This category assesses intellectual impairment, thought disorders, depression, and apathy.
- Part II. Activities of daily living. This category assesses

speech, salivation, swallowing, handwriting, eating, dressing, personal hygiene, turning in bed, falling, freezing when walking, walking, tremors, and sensory complaints such as numbness, tingling, or pain.

- Part III. Motor symptoms. This category assesses speech, facial expression, resting tremor, action tremor, rigidity, finger taps, hand movements, leg agility, rising from a chair, posture, gait, postural stability, and bradykinesia/hypokinesia.
- Part IV. Motor fluctuations. This category assesses the impact of drug therapy on symptoms. It looks at dyskinesias, duration and timing of off and on periods, sleep disturbances, nausea, and orthostasis.

Symptoms are assessed by severity, ranging from 0 (none/normal) to 4 (very severe). The motor fluctuation questions are yes/no answers.

The MDS (Movement Disorders Society) revised the basic UPDRS in 2007, so the version we use today is called the MDS-UPDRS.

The MDS-UPDRS scale is more comprehensive than the Hoehn and Yahr scale or the UPDRS. It's more dynamic, so it's easier to track progress with it. For example, the MDS-UPDRS scale can track if patients improve when they take medication or have surgery to implant a deep brain stimulation device.

The MDS-UPDRS is a more head-to-toe assessment than the Hoehn and Yahr scale. One drawback to this scale is that it's more subjective, because the patient answers a questionnaire for most nonmotor symptoms. For example, the questions about personal hygiene ask the patient, "Over the past week, have you usually been slow or do you need help with washing, bathing, shaving, brushing teeth, combing your hair or with other personal hygiene?" The possible answers are from the patient's own perspective, which may be more positive than what a more objective observer, such as caregiver, might perceive.

The physician or rater part of the MDS-UPDRS has six questions that look at nonmotor symptoms and how they affect the patient's activities of daily living. The questions are designed to cover these areas:

- Cognitive impairment, including bradyphrenia and dementia
- Hallucinations and psychosis
- Depression
- Anxiety
- Apathy
- Compulsive behavior

The response to each question is rated from 0 (none/ normal) to 4 (very severe). The higher the score, the greater the impact of the PD symptoms on the patient.

For all the rating systems, adding up the score tells us whether the patient is trending up (getting worse) or down (improving).

ASSESSING THE PD PATIENT: TECHNIQUES, PEARLS, AND CONSIDERATIONS

THE MOTOR EXAM

Assessing a PD patient takes a head-to-toe examination. The assessment starts with simply observing the patient with a 0 to 4 scale in mind. Is the patient completely normal (0) in terms of facial expression, or is there minimal reduction in expression or animation? This assessment goes up to a score of 4, which is indicative of severe loss of facial expression.

Tremor is an important assessment. With the patient in primary position (seated, legs flat on floor, hands in the lap), we look for tremor at rest. With concentration, many patients can suppress their tremor. An exercise to distract them can unmask the tremor. No tremor is rated 0; severe tremor (10 cm or greater in amplitude) is rated 4. Often, the patient can be distracted from the tremor by closing their eyes and counting backward or subtracting. To test for postural tremor, the patient extends the arms straight out in front.

We also test for kinetic tremor, which is also called movement or action tremor. Have the patient touch their nose with one finger, then reach out to touch the examiner's finger, then repeat back and forth. Look for tremor, especially as the finger nears the nose or the examiner's finger.

It's important to test for all types of tremor because they can overlap or might suggest different disease states.

Next is rigidity. We ask the patient to relax as much as they can, then pick up an arm and move it passively through the joints. Look for a cogwheel motion as the limb moves through the elbow.

If no rigidity is detected with passive motion, we test for rigidity with an activation maneuver that uses rapid alternating movement, such as finger taps on the contralateral side. Often, repeating movements on the contralateral side can unmask rigidity.

Bradykinesia, or slowed movement, can limit a patient's ability to move. To check for it, we note any decrease in amplitude of movement and increase in fatigue when the patient performs repetitive motions.

To test the patient for bradykinesia in the upper extremities, we have them repeatedly tap the thumb and index finger together, first one hand and then the other. Speed of tapping is less important than amplitude. We tell patients,

"I don't care how fast you go; I'm looking to see how big it is." Patients might have normal speed but diminished amplitude or be very slow but have good amplitude. Then test open and close in both hands by having the patients open and close their hands into a fist. This is followed by pronation and supination: palm and dorsum for the hands. Patients go from pronation to supination, front and back. We typically ask them to do this on their lap, as it's a bit more seamless. Again, we look for not only speed but also amplitude.

To test for postural instability, we ask the patient to cross their arms across their chest and stand up. If they can, that rates as 0. On the other end of the scale is the inability to rise at all, which is scored as a 4. Multiple attempts and having to put their hands on the arms of the chair are scored at 2 and 3, respectively.

Testing for postural instability includes gait testing. To test the gait, we ask the patient to stand up and walk across the room and back. As we watch the gait, we're assessing to see how the patient initiates the gait. Does the patient initiate gait by standing up and starting to walk at once, or is there a little bit of hesitation or some small steps before they start moving? The patient may have to rest for a second and then start again.

We note the stride length, which may be diminished or

shuffling. We check the arm swing. The arms should swing steadily, but with PD, one side may swing less. In more advanced PD, both arms may have decreased swing.

Festination, or involuntary acceleration while walking, looks almost like a disconnect between the upper and lower body. The patient speeds up uncontrollably, as if they're running on a down ramp. This can easily lead to falling flat on the face.

We also assess how the patient turns around. Typically, we take two to three steps to turn around, or maybe just one or two when we pivot. Patients with PD have "en bloc" turns. They turn their head, neck, trunk, and pelvis as a rigid unit. They might need anywhere from four steps all the way up to eight steps to turn around.

The next step is testing for retropulsion. We have the patient stand up, then stand behind them and give a little pull backward. Observe how well the patient keeps their balance.

Postural instability can lead to severe falls, bad enough to send the patient to the hospital.

ASSESSING SPEECH AND SWALLOWING

To assess speech, we ask patients to say a sentence such

as "Today is a sunny day" or "The boy caught the dog." By having the patients repeat these, we can judge if the speech is normal or has deteriorated because the PD has advanced. We assign the highest UPDRS speech score (4) when most speech is difficult to understand or unintelligible, with severe volume loss or slurring.

Speech therapy is an extremely important part of patient care. The speech therapist is crucial to the multidisciplinary care team. The Lee Silverman Voice Treatment™ (LSVT) is a specialized form of speech therapy developed specifically for the treatment of PD. It's so important to patients that we'll discuss it in more detail in chapter 5.

Problems with swallowing (dysphagia) are common in PD patients. A swallowing specialist (usually a speech therapist with specialized additional training) can do a swallow test. In the hospital setting, a patient should have a swallowing evaluation early on, especially if they come in with an aspiration-related issue. During a hospitalization, the patient may need to be on a dysphagia diet, with ground or soft foods and thickening agents for liquids.

If a patient is NPO (nothing by mouth) status, it is crucial to continue giving PD medications. At no time should PD drugs ever be withheld. Even if the patient is being prepared for surgery, the PD drugs should still be administered on schedule. They can be given with small sips of water.

DROOLING

Drooling is one of the top symptoms patients complain about, because it's so stigmatizing and disabling. People with PD don't actually overproduce saliva. The drooling happens because they can't efficiently clear it away by swallowing. PD patients lose the innate ability to clear away secretions, so saliva tends to pool up and cause drooling. Hydration to replace the lost liquid is important for patients who have a lot of drooling.

Drooling can be reduced by drugs that dry up the mouth, including the anticholinergic drugs atropine and glycopyrrolate (Robinul), and sometimes by a chemodenervative agent such as botulinum toxins (Botox). Speech therapy with LSVT is extremely helpful for drooling. The therapy works on breathing as much as speech and helps with control of the mouth and lip muscles.

BLOOD PRESSURE FLUCTUATIONS

About 20 percent of patients with Parkinson's will develop problems with blood pressure fluctuations, or orthostatic hypotension. This can lead to not just lightheadedness, dizziness, and nausea upon standing but also falls, confusion, and worsening balance issues.

We recommend checking all hospitalized PD patients for orthostatic hypotension. Measure the blood pressure while the patient is either supine (if possible) or sitting down. Then have them stand up, carefully. Measure again after one minute and again after three minutes. To be sure of picking up orthostatic hypotension, be sure to take the second measurement at three minutes. The patient may not have lost the barostatic reflex after just one minute. After three minutes, however, if they are having trouble maintaining autoregulation, the reflex diminishes. They lose cerebral blood flow and may be at risk of falling.

SLEEP ISSUES

Almost all PD patients have sleep disorders. These often get worse in the inpatient setting, both from the noise and from disruption of usual patterns and often from medications that may promote wakefulness. Nicotine patches and certain antidepressants, such as bupropion (Wellbutrin), for example, promote wakefulness and should be timed to avoid sleep disruption.

To help hospitalized PD patients get enough sleep and avoid worsening their condition, their medications should be reviewed for those that might keep them awake. Both the dose and the timing should be assessed. Stimulating medicines obviously shouldn't be given near bedtime. For example, modafinil (Provigil) or armodafinil (Nuvigil), which are used to counter daytime sleepiness, should be given in the morning as early as possible. If they are administered at or after lunchtime, they can cause insomnia. Similar care should be taken with caffeinated beverages, some asthma inhalers, steroids, selective serotonin reuptake inhibitors (SSRIs), amphetamines and amphetamine-like drugs, and some decongestants.

HOEHN AND YAHR SCORING

Stage 1. Symptoms are very mild; only one side of the body affected (unilateral involvement).

Stage 2. Both sides of the body affected (bilateral involvement), but balance isn't impaired.

Stage 3. Mild to moderate bilateral disease; some postural instability with balance problems, gait disturbances, retropulsion, and increased risk of falls; still physically independent.

Stage 4. Severe disability; cane, walker, or wheelchair may be needed; patient needs help with activities of daily living.

Stage 5. Very debilitated; wheelchair-bound or bedridden.

UPDRS SCORING

Note: Each symptom is assessed on a scale of 0 (none) to 4 (severe). Staging is based on sum of scores.

Part I. Nonmotor aspects of experiences of daily living, including cognitive impairment, hallucinations and psychosis, depression, anxiety, apathy, dopamine dysregulation syndrome, sleep problems, daytime sleepiness, pain and other sensations, urinary problems, constipation, orthostatic hypotension, fatigue

Part II. Motor experiences of daily living, including speech, saliva and drooling, chewing and swallowing, eating tasks, dressing, personal hygiene, handwriting, hobbies and other activities, turning in bed, getting in and out of bed, tremor, walking and balance, freezing

Part III. Motor examination, including speech, facial expression, rigidity, finger tapping, hand movements, toe tapping, leg agility, getting out of chair, gait, freezing, postural stability, posture, bradykinesia, tremor

Part IV. Motor complications, including dyskinesia and motor fluctuations

PART II

TREATMENT

CHAPTER 4

Pharmacological Management

Pharmacological management is the gold standard for treating people with Parkinson's disease. Treatment is symptomatic, with drugs that replace dopamine and relieve some symptoms.

CLASSES OF MEDICATION

Several classes of medications can be used for treating PD. Although the best-known and most prescribed drug is levodopa, drug treatment shouldn't consist of just automatically prescribing it. We take into account many different factors prior to starting the medications. Among the key questions are: What is the road ahead going to be like for this patient? What is the patient's age and psychosocial status? What comorbidities does the patient have?

All factors need to be considered to determine the best treatment options.

LEVODOPA AND CARBIDOPA/LEVODOPA

Up to 90 percent of patients with PD will end up taking levodopa at some point during the duration of their disease. It is the most effective treatment for PD to date.

Levodopa is a precursor to dopamine; it is converted to dopamine in the brain. The drug dopamine itself can't cross the blood-brain barrier, but levodopa can. Levodopa is essentially dopamine in pill form.

Levodopa alone is sometimes prescribed, but most patients do best with a combination tablet containing carbidopa and levodopa (Sinemet, Parcopa). Carbidopa prevents the conversion of levodopa to dopamine. Carbidopa doesn't cross the blood-brain barrier. It inhibits the conversion outside the brain, leaving more levodopa to get into the brain.

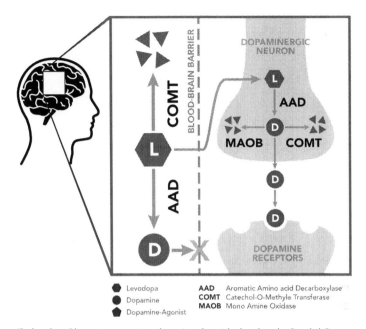

Levodopa	**AAD**	Aromatic Amino acid Decarboxylase
Dopamine	**COMT**	Catechol-O-Methyle Transferase
Dopamine-Agonist	**MAOB**	Mono Amine Oxidase

The levodopa/dopamine enzymatic pathway. Levodopa is broken down by Catechol-O-Methyl Transferase (COMT) and Aromatic Amino Decarboxylase (AAD) outside the blood brain barrier (BBB, dashed lines). Dopamine cannot cross the BBB but Levodopa can. Inside the BBB, Levodopa is converted to Dopamine by AAD. The dopamine is in turn broken down by COMT and also Monoamine Oxidase B (MAOB).

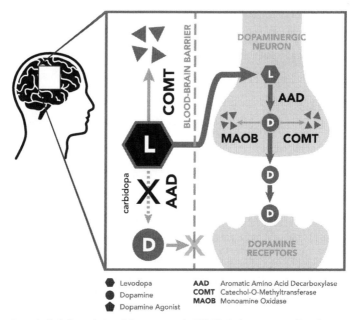

Figure A. Carbidopa which itself does not cross the BBB, blocks the conversion of levodopa to dopamine allowing more levodopa to enter the brain for conversion to dopamine.

Essentially, carbidopa increases the availability of dopamine in the brain. The carbidopa dosage is either 10 mg or 25 mg; the levodopa dosage is 100 mg or 250 mg. For lower doses of levodopa, the tablet can be cut in half. The range of possible doses makes using this drug more dynamic. The best preparation and dosage for each patient must be individually determined. As a rule of thumb when initiating levodopa, we start with a low dose and titrate up progressively.

Rytary Carbidopa/Levodopa Extended-Release Capsules

Rytary is an extended-release form of carbidopa/levodopa that has a duration of effect of about five to eight hours. The capsule contains the drugs in three different types of beads. The first kick in within about an hour, the second set lasts about five to eight hours, and the third set has tartaric acid, which helps enhance absorption. Rytary is available in four different strengths and provides additional treatment options beyond Sinemet.

Duopa Carbidopa/Levodopa Enteric Suspension

Some patients with advanced PD who can no longer swallow or who have absorption problems in the GI tract can have carbidopa/levodopa delivered by pump directly to the jejunum in the small intestine. The formulation for this is a suspension called Duopa. It's delivered continuously into the intestine over 16 hours through a tube attached to a small portable pump. To receive Duopa, the patient has a procedure to place the PEG-J tube.

Pump delivery avoids GI tract absorption problems and provides much smoother plasma delivery of levodopa. Duopa is fairly new on the market and isn't appropriate for most patients with advanced disease—most can't handle the complexity of using the pump.

ADHERENCE TO TIMING OF PARKINSON'S MEDICATIONS IS CRITICAL.

The timing of drug administration isn't really because

of its half-life. Half-life clearance refers to the clearance from the blood. While, in general, half-life can be correlated to clearance of efficacy in a patient without PD, PD patients are different. Patients who have had Parkinson's for a long time have stunted responses to these medications, so they require increasingly large doses that are independent of the chemical half-life in the body. In these patients, the efficacy of the drug becomes more short-lived and erratic, independent of the chemical half-life.

This erratic efficacy of the medication in PD patients results in what we call motor fluctuation. It means patients fluctuate or cycle between "on" time (when medications are efficacious) and "off" time (when they don't work). In patients who have been on medication for a longer period, this cycling happens multiple times during the day. For these patients, medications are administered in higher doses and also closer intervals. Higher doses of levodopa are in turn associated with higher chances of motor fluctuation and dyskinesias, no matter what preparation is prescribed. (Dyskinesias are uncontrollable writhing movements of the head, mouth, extremities, or trunk that occur as a side effect of higher doses of medications.)

Although levodopa is the most effective drug for PD, it's not necessarily the first medication that should be used. We take the patient's age, comorbidities, psychosocial status, and the road ahead of them into account when deciding to start levodopa. The important ELLDOPA study in 2004 showed that higher doses can lead to motor complications early on.

A hospitalized PD patient may not be comfortable with starting on a higher dose of levodopa. Instead, as part of discharge planning, arrange a consultation with a movement disorders specialist if at all possible.

After taking a dose of Sinemet IR (instant release), the typical time to onset is about 15 to 30 minutes. In advanced cases, onset will take longer. When patients first start taking this drug, the duration of effect is up to six to eight hours. We call this the honeymoon period, because patients respond quickly and often dramatically. As the disease progresses, however, the time to onset gets longer, the dose gets larger, and the effect gets smaller.

When patients start using levodopa, they do really well. They might only need three doses a day. They feel like it keeps them on; they have fewer symptoms or none at all. They usually have those six to eight hours of feeling really good.

As the disease advances and patients lose more and more dopamine neurons, that window starts to close. The drug takes longer to kick in, and the "on" window diminishes. It might go from six hours to only three. The effect wears off quicker. As the disease advances even more, the on window gets so small that the drug takes anywhere from 60 to 90 minutes to start working and the effect might last for only two to three hours or even less. Long before that point, the patient is already experiencing dyskinesia, or abnormal movements, caused by the drug. The threshold for dyskinesia gets lower as that window gets smaller. The movement disorders neurologist spends much time with these patients and their caregivers, adjusting the medication and fine-tuning the timing to minimize motor fluctuations, off times, and dyskinesias. The patients become very dependent on the timing, and any deviations from their regimen can cause significant setbacks.

Levodopa primarily helps with motor symptoms, but it often also improves other symptoms, such as sleep disturbances.

Levodopa should not be given based simply on the standard hospital nursing schedule of TID or QID. If a patient should get levodopa four times a day, it should be given at the times the patient or patient's caregiver says they usually take it. The intervals may not be regular and may seem illogical or incorrect, but whatever schedule has been working for the patient is the schedule to follow. For patients with more advanced PD, that schedule was painstakingly worked out to try to minimize motor fluctuations, off times, and the side effects of the medication.

Disrupting it will cause additional problems for the hospitalized patient. We have to follow the patient's schedule, not the hospital's.

We have to ensure consistency with the timing; a delay of even 15 minutes can cause a patient to be off. In addition, we have to make sure the correct formulation is administered to the patient. If a patient is on regular Sinemet, they should not be placed on Sinemet CR or ER, as this can have the same deleterious effect of missing a dose. The exception to this is if a patient is unable to swallow. An immediate-release dose, which can be crushed, can be used to replace extended-release Sinemet, which cannot be crushed. We do this simply to allow the administration of some medication.

NPO status for a PD patient should be challenged with regard to medication. It is crucially important for patients to get their medication on time and not miss any doses.

PD patients need their meds just to be able to move. Withholding them because of NPO status only worsens their condition and can lead to a patient becoming frozen. Most PD drugs can be crushed and given in applesauce or pudding. In fact, Rytary capsules are designed to be opened and sprinkled on food. When in doubt about crushing an extended-release drug, substitute the regular form instead of skipping the dose. If the drug is not available on the formulary or it's unavailable in general, check with the patient's caregiver. Hospitals often have policies that allow patients to bring medications from home.

MEDICATION ADMINISTRATION FOR NPO PATIENTS

MEDICATION	ADMINISTRATION
Sinemet standard release	Can be crushed and dissolved in applesauce. Can be dispersed in water for one to five minutes to be placed into G-tubes.
Sinemet CR	Should not be crushed. Should be converted to standard release if patient is unable to swallow. Because Sinemet standard release has a quicker onset and shorter duration of action, consider dividing the CR dose to two standard-release doses. For example, instead of Sinemet CR 25-100 every four hours, consider giving regular Sinemet 25-100, half a tab every two hours.
Requip	Can be crushed and dissolved in water or applesauce.
Mirapex	Can be crushed and dissolved in water or applesauce.
Rytary	Capsule can be opened and sprinkled over applesauce.
Entacapone	Can be crushed and dissolved in applesauce. Can be dissolved in water for feeding tubes.
Stalevo	Do not crush. This drug is a combination of carbidopa/levodopa/entacapone. It can be converted to carbidopa/levodopa standard release plus entacapone. These can be crushed and dissolved in applesauce. The most common doses of Stalevo are 100 mg, 150 mg, or 200 mg, which is also the levodopa component. They all have 200 mg of entacapone.
Amantadine	Open capsule and dissolve in water.
Rasagiline	Can be crushed and dissolved in water or applesauce.
Selegiline	Can be crushed and dissolved in water or applesauce.

The above is based on personal experience, with some pharma suggestions and available literature. We strongly recommend discussing these with your hospital pharmacy.

Levodopa Side Effects

Nausea, dizziness, dry mouth, GI disturbances, and rashes are common side effects of levodopa. When the doses get higher as the disease progresses, side effects such as confusion and hallucinations can occur. Levodopa can also cause eye blinking/twitching, impulse control disorders, mood changes (depression), and worsening of dyskinesia.

Keeping the patient on the same levodopa formulation during a hospitalization is extremely important. In the hospital, if a drug isn't on the formulary, either the pharmacy or the electronic medical system may suggest an alternative. PD medications should not be interchanged, even for drugs that may be in the same class or have a similar mechanism of action. Again, the drug regimen for an advanced PD patient has been very carefully customized. Replacing the patient's medication with what's available at the hospital is not adequate. In these situations, the options are to request that nonformulary medication be given to the patient or to ask the patient, or family members or caregivers, to bring the patient's own medication to the hospital.

Always keep the patient on whatever they're already using. Be thoughtful and meticulous about the differences and preparations; these drugs are not interchangeable.

The medications a PD patient is taking have been prescribed meticulously, with a lot of thought. When patients are admitted, it's vital not to scramble the drugs by switching to a different formulation or substituting drugs that appear similar but actually have different mechanisms of action.

INVOLVING CAREGIVERS

The patient or the patient's caregiver is the best source of guidance for the levodopa dosing schedule. They probably know a lot more than the staff doctor about how the patient responds to a drug and when the best time to take it is. The caregiver may not always be there when a patient is hospitalized, however. It's important to proactively reach out, especially if a patient is in the emergency room or admitted emergently. Reach out to the family member or caregiver and get a really good history. For these patients, history is everything, especially for medication timing, the exact formulations, and adverse effects. The caregiver can tell you if the patient routinely takes a drug crushed in applesauce, for instance, and the best times for dosing. The role of the caregiver in taking a patient's history is equal to, if not more important than, the patient's. Nothing beats a good history.

DOPAMINE AGONISTS

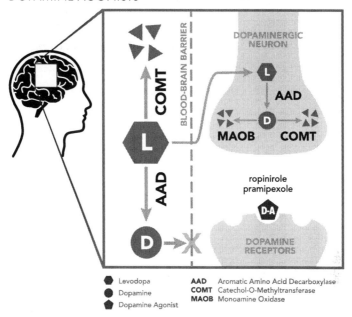

Figure B. Dopamine agonists work by activating post synaptic dopamine receptors.

Dopamine agonists work by stimulating the dopamine receptors in the brain. These drugs can be used as monotherapy or as adjunctive therapy with levodopa. Dopamine agonists may help to smooth out the on/off effect of levodopa. As with monoamine oxidase B (MAO-B) inhibitors, they are a good choice for younger patients who want to avoid levodopa for as long as possible. They're helpful for younger patients who are more symptomatic, with moderate tremor, bradykinesia, or rigidity. These people need more than an MAO-B inhibitor but aren't ready for levodopa yet.

The side effects of dopamine agonists have to be considered. Nausea and lightheadedness are common side effects. Sleep attacks may happen, especially when the patient first starts taking the drug. Some swelling and irritation at the injection site can occur (with injectable versions). Some patients will develop impulse control disorders, such as compulsive gambling or shopping, from these drugs. This is a serious concern—we've seen patients end up in the hospital because of drug-related impulsiveness or compulsivity.

Dopamine agonists come in several different types:

- Apomorphine (Apokyn, Ixense, Spontane, Uprima). Injected subcutaneously as needed, using injector pen.
- Pramipexole (Mirapex, Mirapex ER). Tablets.
- Ropinirole (Requip and Requip XL). Tablets.
- Rotigotine (Neupro). Once-daily transdermal patch. Very helpful for patients with dysphagia.

Older dopamine agonists, such as bromocriptine, pergolide, and cabergoline, increased the risk of heart problems and are now only rarely prescribed. The dopamine agonists used today do not have an increased risk of heart damage.

Finding the optimal dose of a dopamine agonist takes

some time. Simply starting a patient on a dopamine agonist isn't good enough. Close follow-up is needed to determine the optimal dose that balances efficacy with side effects. This often requires multiple dose adjustments. Patients shouldn't adjust their medication on their own; they should work with their doctor, physician assistant, or nurse.

For any concerns regarding the doses of medications, arrange for a movement disorders consult. At the least, arrange a conversation with the patient's own movement disorders neurologist.

Inpatients should be closely observed to note if the effect of a drug seems to be less strong than it was previously. Every patient is different and has different doses, but dose titration may be needed, especially if PD symptoms appear worse upon admission.

EMERGING DOPAMINE THERAPIES

A number of PD drugs are in the approval pipeline. An inhaled version of levodopa, with a fast time to onset, may be available soon. The levodopa is inhaled with a mask and enters the bloodstream directly instead of passing through the gut.

The injected dopamine promoter apomorphine (Apokyn)

may soon be available in a sublingual (placed under the tongue) form, with a fast onset of action. Patch forms of levodopa are in the works, and so are additional pump forms.

OTHER CLASSES OF MEDICATIONS

Several other classes of medication can be helpful for PD. They can be used on their own (monotherapy) or in conjunction with levodopa.

MAO-B INHIBITORS

MAO-B is an enzyme that breaks down dopamine in the cells. MAO-B inhibitors keep the enzyme from breaking down dopamine so that there's more of it in the brain and its action is prolonged.

Some data show these drugs can be used by themselves to boost dopamine levels in the brain. That makes this class of drugs a good choice for treating younger patients with early onset PD. They're going to be on drugs for a long time, so the longer we can help their symptoms without going to levodopa, the more we can delay the inevitable side effects that come with it.

MAO-B inhibitors are probably the best tolerated of all PD drugs.

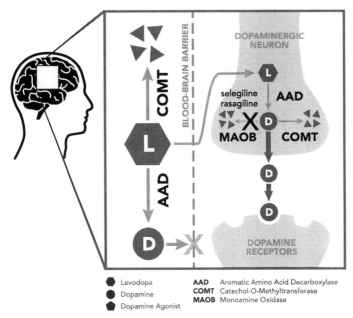

● Levodopa	**AAD**	Aromatic Amino Acid Decarboxylase
● Dopamine	**COMT**	Catechol-O-Methyltransferase
⬠ Dopamine Agonist	**MAOB**	Monoamine Oxidase

Figure C. MAOB inhibitors reduce the breakdown of dopamine in the neurons by blocking the enzyme monoamine oxidase B (MAOB).

They're a good adjunctive therapy for levodopa. These drugs come in several different types:

- Selegiline (Eldepryl, Atapryl, Carbex). This was one of the first MAO-Bs to become available; it dates back to the 1980s. It's typically taken twice a day. Because selegiline can break down into an amphetamine metabolite, the timing for taking the medication is important. We've seen patients take this drug at 6:00 p.m. and then not be able to sleep. For hospitalized patients, try to give both doses before 2:00 p.m. (with breakfast and lunch).
- Selegiline (Zydis). The sublingual form of selegiline.

- Rasagiline (Azilect). Typically taken once daily. This drug does not break down into an amphetamine.

MAO-B inhibitors can cause nausea, joint pain, trouble sleeping, and lightheadedness. They can also cause sudden daytime sleepiness, or sleep attacks. In rare cases, they can cause a dangerous rise in blood pressure. The side effect that bothers patients the most is that MAO-B inhibitors can worsen the dyskinesia caused by levodopa, because now more dopamine is available in the brain to patients who are already prone to dyskinesia. We can adjust the levodopa dose downward to compensate.

MAO-B inhibitors can also interact with a number of drugs, including meperidine (Demerol) and dextromethorphan (used for cough suppression). Rasagiline (Azilect) interacts with ciprofloxacin (Cipro). If the patient needs surgery, the anesthesiologist should be aware of the MAO-B use. The herbal supplement St. John's wort may also have an interaction with MAO-B inhibitors.

To prevent a serious high blood pressure reaction while taking MAO-B inhibitors, patients need to avoid eating foods high in the amino acid tyramine. Foods high in tyramine include aged cheeses, dried or aged meats and sausages such as salami, preserved fish such as pickled herring, fermented foods such as sauerkraut and kimchi, and soy foods such as soy sauce and tofu. Beer and red wine also should be avoided. Even foods with moderate amounts of tyramine, including avocados, bananas, eggplant, green beans, raisins, raspberries, red plums, spinach, tomatoes, chocolate, yogurt, sour cream, peanuts, coffee, cola, distilled spirits, and white wine, should be limited. For hospitalized patients, arrange for a dietitian to review the restrictions. Many patients don't like the limits on alcohol. It's important to counsel them about why they need to avoid some forms of alcohol and limit others.

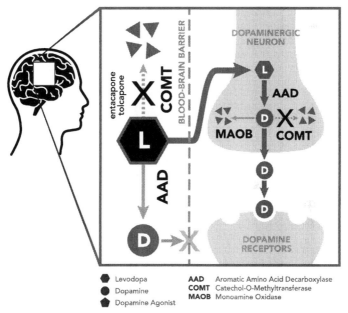

Figure D. COMT breaks down dopamine in the neurons and also levodopa outside the blood brain barrier. COMT inhibitors increase the availability of dopamine by inhibiting this enzyme's activity.

COMT INHIBITORS

COMT inhibitors block the action of the enzyme catechol-O-methyltransferase, which breaks down levodopa. Blocking this enzyme makes the effects of levodopa last longer. COMT inhibitors aren't monotherapy. They only work when given with levodopa or levodopa/carbidopa. They're most effective when the patient has been taking a levodopa dose of 600 mg or less without dyskinesia and is experiencing symptoms as the drug wears off. COMT inhibitors help smooth out the effects as levodopa wears off.

Several different COMT inhibitors are available:

- Entacapone (Comtan). One tablet taken up to eight times a day.
- Carbidopa/levodopa with entacapone (Stalevo). One tablet taken up to eight times a day.
- Tolcapone (Tasmar). One tablet taken three times a day.

The side effects of COMT inhibitors include dizziness, nausea, lightheadedness, and sleep disturbances. They may make dyskinesia symptoms worse until the dose is adjusted. Tolcapone can cause serious, even fatal, liver damage. Patients taking this drug must be carefully monitored. For this reason, it isn't commonly prescribed in the United States.

AMANTADINE

Amantadine is thought to work in the brain through multiple, but not-well-understood, mechanisms. It is an NMDA antagonist and is thought to increase dopamine release and block dopamine reuptake. When this drug was first prescribed back in the 1950s, it was to treat influenza. Doctors and patients noted that it also helped dyskinesia and tremor, so it entered the PD pharmacology. It can be helpful for treating tremor and for reducing levodopa-induced dyskinesia, although there's not a lot of data to support this. It may be prescribed as a first-line therapy if the patient has severe tremors. Amantadine takes several weeks to start working, and the benefit may not last for more than six months or so.

Amantadine isn't a benign drug, however, especially for older patients. It can have a lot of side effects, including hallucinations, confusion, dry mouth, and a rash called livedo reticularis (mottled, purplish rash, often seen on the legs or torso). Any of these symptoms means it's time to discontinue the drug.

The extended-release form of amantadine (Gocovri) was approved in 2017.

TRIHEXYPHENIDYL

Trihexyphenidyl or trihexy (Artane) is an anticholinergic

(drug that blocks the neurotransmitter acetylcholine in the nervous system). It is a very old drug for PD that isn't used much now. The primary use is as a monotherapy to treat tremor, but it can also be given in conjunction with levodopa.

Keep clinical considerations and side effects in mind, including dry eyes, dry mouth, fast or irregular heartbeat, anxiety, hallucinations, confusion, agitation, and a slow heart rate for older patients.

OTHER MEDICATIONS

People with PD may need additional medication to treat related and unrelated health issues. Most commonly used drugs are safe, but doctors and hospital, rehab, and nursing home staff need to be very aware that some drugs are contraindicated for people taking drugs to treat PD symptoms.

ANTIPSYCHOTICS

Antipsychotics may be prescribed for a patient who is starting to hallucinate, is having impulsivity, or is aggressive, agitated, or combative. This class of medication should be carefully considered and avoided if at all possible in PD patients. Many antipsychotics can make their Parkinsonism symptoms worse and cause drowsiness or confusion.

Antipsychotic medications can block dopamine receptors, which can make a patient with PD more prone to tremor, rigidity, bradykinesia, and gait disturbances. Although these drugs aren't absolutely contraindicated, they should be used with caution. This is particularly true of older antipsychotics such as haloperidol (Haldol) and chlorpromazine (Thorazine).

Atypical antipsychotics have less direct dopaminergic blockade. Drugs such as quetiapine (Seroquel) or clozapine (Clorazil) may be used in some patients.

A new antipsychotic drug called pimavanserin (Nuplazid) was approved in 2016 by the Food and Drug Administration (FDA). Pimavanserin is the only drug indicated specifically for PD psychosis. It has no dopaminergic action. Because it takes anywhere from four to eight weeks to kick in, pimavanserin won't usually be started in a hospital setting, but it may be considered for outpatient use.

ANTIEMETICS

Some antiemetics for GI problems such as nausea work in ways similar to the neuroleptic drugs. The drugs metoclopramide (Reglan) and domperidone (Motilium) help with gastroparesis and work by blocking dopamine and should be avoided in patients with PD. Metoclopramide can cause dizziness, drowsiness, and insomnia and can make dyskinesias worse. It can also interact with a long list of drugs. Domperidone can cause cardiac arrhythmias, cardiac arrest, and sudden death. It has not been widely prescribed in the United States because its use was restricted by the FDA in 2004. Exceptions are made, however, for patients with severe GI motility disorders who haven't been helped by other drugs.

PAIN MEDICATION

Most standard pain medications are safe for PD patients. Narcotic medications may cause confusion or psychosis, however. Narcotic medications can also cause constipation, which is already a problem for almost all PD patients. Use these drugs cautiously and always initiate use of a stool softener at the same time. Prescribe anti-inflammatories and non-narcotics instead whenever possible. Patients on selegiline should not be given meperidine (Demerol).

ANTIDEPRESSANTS

Depression, anxiety, and apathy are very common non-motor symptoms of PD. People with Parkinson's have abnormally low levels of the neurotransmitter GABA (gamma-Aminobutyric acid), which affects the same brain pathways as anxiety and depression. Antianxiety medications designed to increase GABA levels can be very helpful. Anxiety is sometimes directly linked to fluctuations in motor symptoms. During off periods, patients can become severely anxious or even have anxiety attacks.

Depression is part of PD—at least half of all PD patients will experience it. Depression in PD is caused by changes in brain chemistry in the areas of the brain that produce dopamine, norepinephrine, and serotonin. These chemicals help regulate mood, energy, motivation, and sleep. Depression can make motor and nonmotor symptoms worse. Physicians and caregivers should be alert for signs of depression and not ignore or undertreat it. Treating depression can improve movement and the patient's quality of life.

Antidepressant drugs can be a big help. The selective serotonin reuptake inhibitors (SSRIs), antidepressants, such as fluoxetine (Prozac), sertraline (Zoloft), paroxetine (Paxil), citalopram (Celexa), and escitalopram (Lexapro), are all safe to use. Monitor patients on MAO-B inhibitors for interactions, however.

Tricyclic antidepressants may also be used. Serotonin-norepinephrine reuptake inhibitors (SNRIs) such as desvenlafaxine (Pristiq, Khedezla), duloxetine (Cymbalta), venlafaxine (Effexor), and levomilnacipran (Fetzima) are safe. Amoxapine (Asendin) should not be used.

Counsel patients and caregivers that all these medications may take some time to work. Be sure to prescribe adequate dosing and explain the importance of continuing to take the drug. Hospitalized patients should continue to take their antidepressants.

Electroconvulsive therapy (ECT) is considered safe. It is sometimes an option for patients with PD suffering from depression. We've had patients use it successfully when antidepressant drugs didn't help.

DRUG CONSIDERATIONS

THE LEVODOPA "ON WINDOW"

When patients start taking levodopa, they usually do very well—at first. The drug will kick in in less than 30 minutes, the "on" effect can last from five up to eight hours, and then the drug will wear off gently.

As time goes on, the "on window," the period when the drug has efficacy and predictability, gets smaller and smaller. The medication takes longer to work. Instead of kicking in within 30 minutes, it might be 30 to 60 minutes. The on time can shorten to only maybe four hours. The dose wears off abruptly, and the patient can unpredictably turn "off."

Eventually, patients can start having dose failures, where

the medication fails to work, or they experience unpredictable offs, where the on time suddenly drops from perhaps four hours to only two. The threshold for developing dyskinesias decreases. The patient might be on but have dyskinesias, which are very disabling abnormal involuntary movements.

Healthcare providers need to be aware of these phenomena and realize that a patient may fluctuate in mobility. Activities can be scheduled keeping this in mind.

Off periods can have a myriad of symptoms that go beyond just tremors, muscle cramps, dystonia, or sensory disturbances. Even anxiety and shortness of breath can occur in the off state. When off symptoms start to appear, that indicates it's time for another dose, even if it might be off the patient's schedule.

SIDE EFFECTS AND THE BENEFIT-VERSUS-RISK EQUATION

Even when it's been initially started and is working well, levodopa can cause some short-term side effects, such as nausea, dizziness, edema, and confusion. Eventually, as the on-window narrows, levodopa causes motor fluctuations and dyskinesias.

The long-term effects can take years to kick in. Every patient with PD is different, but on average, on and off periods of motor fluctuations start to develop within three to five years after starting levodopa.

Because every patient is different, so are the drug regimes. Each patient's regimen is assessed, adjusted, and reassessed over time to maximize the benefits and reduce the side effects. The dosing interval, the time during the day when medication is started, and the choice of medication take much trial and effort to fine-tune, working with the patient, caregivers, and the movement disorders specialist.

This is why it is so important to pay attention to the medication regimen when patients are admitted to the hospital. To avoid difficulties for the patient in regard to their Parkinson's symptoms, the carefully designed medication regimen must be followed closely.

Communicating directly and clearly with the patients, family, and caretakers is crucial. No two people with Parkinson's are alike. For healthcare providers, that means understanding the medication history is paramount. We need to know the right doses and exact timing of medications. We have to be meticulous when taking this history. Sometimes a patient being admitted to the hospital is confused and may not be able to provide a good medication history. If any doubt exists, we should seek out family members and caregivers to try to supplement the history.

DRUGS FOR PD

DRUG CLASS	GENERIC NAME	BRAND NAME
Levodopa	carbidopa/levodopa	Sinemet, Rytary, Duopa
Monoamine oxidase inhibitors	selegiline	Eldepryl, Atapryl, Carbex
	rasagiline	Azilect
Dopamine agonists	apomorphine	Apokyn, Ixense, Spontane, Uprima
	pramipexole	Mirapex
	ropinirole	Requip
	rotigotine	Neupro
COMT Inhibitors	entacapone	Comtan
	carbidopa/levodopa with entacapone	Stalevo
	tolcapone	Tasmar
NMDA receptor agonist	amantadine	Gocovri
Anticholinergic	trihexyphenidyl	Artane

SURGICAL TREATMENT

Deep brain stimulation (DBS) is a therapy that can offer relief of some symptoms of PD. This therapy involves implanting electrodes in the brain that are attached to a pacemaker, which is often implanted subclavicularly, very similar to a cardiac pacemaker. Not everyone is a surgical candidate, and as the surgery offers symptomatic treatment for only some motor symptoms of PD, the selection process is rigorous to ensure proper identification of patients who will benefit most from the therapy.

DBS offers relief for tremors, rigidity, and bradykinesia

associated with PD. In addition, it can improve motor fluctuations and allows some medication reduction.

Gait and balance do not respond well to DBS, nor do nonmotor symptoms. In the correctly selected patient, however, the therapy can significantly improve quality of life.

While a detailed discussion of DBS is beyond the scope of this book, it is important to have some familiarity with the therapy and its implications in the hospital setting.

DBS therapy is always on and is chronic stimulation, in comparison to a heart pacemaker, which is an "as-needed therapy." It is not common that patients in the hospital need adjustments to the DBS therapy; however, if a patient is admitted with an acutely changed exam, it is important to ensure the device is on and properly functioning.

Most large hospitals will have a team with expertise in DBS that can help identify if there are any issues with the device. The representative from the manufacturer should also always be able to assist in addressing these concerns.

What If a Patient with DBS Needs a Test?

Patients who have DBS may undergo most tests without any issues. Any procedure requiring an electrocardiogram (EKG) may need the device to be turned off simply because of the electrical artifact for the EKG caused by the stimulation. Most patients are able to turn their device off for the procedure; however, if there is any concern, representatives of the manufacturer can be contacted to facilitate. Currently, only two companies have FDA-approved devices that are available in US markets. They are Medtronic Neuromodulation Inc. and Abbott Scientific (formerly St. Jude). Contact information for both is provided at the end this section and at the end of the book.

What If a Patient with DBS Needs to Undergo Surgery?

During surgery, Medtronic recommends turning the device off, and Abbott has a "surgery mode" that can be turned on easily by the patient or, if needed, a representative from the manufacturer.

What about Magnetic Resonance Imaging (MRI)?

Patients can undergo most imaging with DBS. MRI is permitted by Medtronic and will likely be permitted by Abbott as well at the time of release of this book; however, certain guidelines and protocols have to be followed, which can be guided by the manufacturer.

Other Concerns

Any other concerns with the devices can be referred to the manufacturer. They are very responsive, and answers can usually be obtained fairly quickly.

Medtronic Neuromodulation Patient Services: 1-800-510-6735

Abbott Scientific Technical Support: 1-800-727-7846, option 3

CHAPTER 5

Nonmotor Parkinson's Disease Symptoms in the Hospital

People with Parkinson's disease experience more than just motor fluctuations or tremor. They have symptoms that can't be corrected by levodopa and drugs that affect dopamine. The range of other symptoms is very large. Every patient presents with different symptoms and progresses differently. We can help these patients best by being aware of the wide range of possible symptoms and, if needed, assembling a multidisciplinary team for diagnosis and treatment. Managing symptoms effectively benefits the patient's quality of life and ability to remain independent and can also make hospitalizations less traumatic.

SLEEP DISORDERS

Adequate, good-quality sleep is very important for patients with PD. Sleep is important for neurorestoration in the brain. When these patients don't sleep well, they're more prone to worsening symptomology, including cognitive disturbances and delirium. In the hospital, patients often have difficulty sleeping because of the unfamiliar surroundings, ongoing noise, and the routine disruptions by staff performing needed tasks. In addition, many patients already have a disrupted sleep-wake cycle, with sleep fragmentation, rapid eye movement behavior disorder (REMBD), and often also nocturia.

To help patients sleep better in the hospital, we try to keep to their usual medication schedule. Some drugs cause wakefulness and should not be given in the late afternoon or evening.

We prefer to try nonpharmacological approaches first before resorting to sleep drugs. Educating patients on proper sleep hygiene is important. A cool, dark room with no TV is a standard recommendation for patients having trouble falling asleep at home. In the hospital, avoiding noise and disruption of sleep is difficult, but some steps can be taken to help improve the environment. Placing patients with PD away from the nurses' station on a quieter part of the floor can help. Making sure they get their evening Parkinson's medications on time can be essential.

Many patients need dopamine to get through the night in terms of mobility and being able to move in bed. Missing the evening dose or delaying it can have profound effects on sleep.

If sleep agents are needed, we recommend a long-acting benzodiazepine, such as clonazepam (Klonopin), because of its long half-life. Other benzodiazepines (Ativan, Valium, Xanax, and many others) may be used, but they are not as effective. The hormone melatonin may also be helpful for sleep. Frequent urination at night (nocturia) can often disrupt sleep. An anticholinergic drug such as oxybutynin (Oxytrol), tolterodine (Detrol), trospium (Regurin, Sanctura), solifenacin (Vesicare), or mirabegron (Myrbetriq) given at bedtime may minimize urinary episodes at night. Practitioners must be aware of potential cognitive side effects from these drugs, particularly if the patient has not had a trial prior to hospitalization.

We recommend avoiding drugs such as zolpidem (Ambien) and eszopiclone (Lunesta). While these drugs will put a patient to sleep, they won't help them stay asleep. They can also exacerbate some preexisting issues and can exacerbate confusion.

Where possible, we recommend napping during the day to help PD patients catch up on sleep.

AUTONOMIC CHANGES

Common autonomic changes include excessive sweating, constipation, urinary issues, and neurogenic orthostatic hypotension.

Many patients will end up in the hospital because of neurogenic orthostatic hypotension, which is a drop in blood pressure of 20 mm mercury systolic or 10 mm mercury diastolic as the patient moves from lying or sitting to standing. The large drop in blood pressure can cause nausea, lightheadedness, dizziness, and falls. Even disorientation and trouble breathing can occur at times.

The problem can be minimized in the hospital by elevating the head of the bed 10 to 15 degrees. Patients should be cautious about standing up too quickly. They should sit on the side of the bed for a minute or two before rising. Physical therapists should teach their patients how to use gradual movements to stand up and should be aware of potential blood pressure fluctuations.

Adequate hydration helps, as does liberalizing salt intake. Compression stockings with an abdominal binder may also be used to minimize venous pooling and help prevent orthostasis.

If medication is needed because of continued issues with orthostatic hypotension, the options are fludrocortisone

(Florinef), midodrine (Amatine, ProAmatine), and droxidopa (Northera).

PD patients, by definition, are at risk for falls and should
wear fall-risk bracelets. In the hospital, rehab, and nursing home, bed alarms should be used even if orthostatic
hypotension isn't a problem.

PSYCHIATRIC SYMPTOMS

As discussed in chapter 3, depression, apathy, anxiety,
and psychosis are all common psychiatric symptoms of
PD. While it is not realistic to address these disorders
when patients are in the hospital for non-PD reasons, it
is important to be familiar with them, how they can affect
PD patients, and the higher prevalence of these disorders
in PD patients than those without PD.

ANXIETY

Anxiety affects upward of 40 to 50 percent of Parkinson's
patients. It can be episodic or more frequent; it can also
present as panic attacks. Obtaining a thorough history of
anxiety, including medications, can be very helpful. Especially before stressful situations happen in the hospital,
understanding the patient's response to anxiety helps
address the patient better and more effectively. Benzodiazepine drugs can be helpful.

APATHY

Apathy is a very common nonmotor symptom in PD patients. Apathy can also be a symptom of depression unrelated to PD. A patient who appears to be apathetic should be assessed by a mental health professional with experience in PD to determine how much of the apathy is related to depression and how much is inherent to PD. If the apathy is depression-related, it should be treated. Parkinson's patients with inherent apathy need continuous encouragement to be active and engaged. Sometimes increasing the levodopa dose helps. While it is difficult to discern these subtleties in the hospital setting, it is important to be aware of the possibility of apathy in a PD patient who may not want to participate in prescribed activities in the hospital such as physical therapy. Gentle but continuous encouragement may be fruitful in these instances.

PSYCHOSIS: HALLUCINATIONS AND DELIRIUM

Psychosis often develops in Parkinson's patients as the disease progresses. It can be very disabling. It's a common reason for hospitalization and can often result in the family being unable to care for the patient and placing them in a nursing home. Psychosis can also manifest as paranoia or delusions, especially persecutory delusions.

Psychosis and delirium can occur in the hospital and they

can complicate the care of PD patients. Healthcare practitioners should be familiar with their occurrence and know some strategies for treatment.

Psychosis can be exacerbated in the hospital if PD medications are delayed or if contraindicated medications are administered.

Psychosis is important to define and treat. In the hospital or rehab facility, environment is key. Noise and other stressors can exacerbate it. Some patients experience sundowning in which symptoms worsen in the evening.

If psychosis or delirium occurs in a PD patient, avoid medications such as haloperidol (Haldol) or other typical antipsychotics, as they can worsen PD symptoms.

An atypical antipsychotic such as quetiapine (Seroquel) is better tolerated by PD patients and can be effective. Other antipsychotics can be used in the PD population but starting them in the hospital setting may not be ideal. Some, such as clozapine (Clozaril), have potential side effects; others, such as pimavanserin (Nuplazid), take some time to be effective. Clozapine requires blood monitoring and can cause significant weight gain; it can also cause a rare but potentially fatal agranulocytosis. Pimavanserin is an antipsychotic drug designed specifically to help with hallucinations for people with PD. It was approved in 2016. This drug is effective, but it takes several weeks to work.

Hallucinations can be common for patients who have had PD for a long time. When a patient hallucinates, the caregiver's first response should be to define the nature of the hallucination and to determine if the patient has retained insight. Is the patient aware of the hallucination? Does the patient know that what they're experiencing isn't real? People who retain insight usually manage hallucinations well, without getting too upset by them. When insight is lost, however, these patients tend to do worse and are more difficult to manage.

Every patient is different and needs to be assessed individually. There are no firm guidelines for dealing with hallucinations in PD patients.

Patients who are hallucinating are helped if a caregiver reassures them and gently reminds them that what they're seeing (or hearing or smelling or feeling) isn't really there. If the patient has retained insight, this is reassuring. If the patient has lost insight and responds to the hallucination as if it were real, they often get very distressed. Reminding the patient kindly of what's real, and not just saying, "That's not there" or "I don't know what you're talking about" will often suffice. Be gentle. Let them work through it. If reassurance doesn't help, medications may need to be considered instead.

Hallucinations can be unpleasant or frightening, but not always. We have some patients who see late loved ones and don't find the experience distressing. Another patient may just see little children and not experience any unpleasant hallucinations.

Patients with psychosis may get physical and lash out. Avoid restraint if at all possible, because that only agitates them more and leads to a vicious circle of anti-psychotic drugs and more restraint. Use caution when giving agitated patients intramuscular injections; take this approach only if they absolutely need it. Additionally, confer with team members in neurology and psychiatry to determine what the best plan of action may be.

Parkinson's patients may be prone to delirium in the hospital setting, particularly if they have already been dealing with psychosis. Delirium doesn't occur often in outpatients. The noisy, confusing hospital environment and lack of sleep can cause delirium, but other causes, such as infection or an underlying history of dementia, should be ruled out first. A thorough evaluation should be done to look for a precipitating cause. In distinguishing between delirium and psychosis, delirium is more acute.

The delirium usually lasts for a much shorter time than dementia or psychosis.

During delirium, patients may be agitated and impulsive—they may try to get out of bed when they really need to stay there, for example.

Some evidence shows that patients with PD who are admitted to the hospital may experience delirium if PD medications are delayed. This is a recurring theme throughout this book: attention to timing is crucial in PD medications.

Delirium is another example of why multidisciplinary care is so important. The patient's team should include a psychiatrist and/or a neurologist. When guidance is needed for treating these patients, these team members can help.

ENTERIC ISSUES

GI issues are common among PD patients. Constipation is the most common symptom.

CONSTIPATION

Constipation is very distressing for patients. It can be an early symptom of PD, sometimes occurring years before a diagnosis is made. As the disease progresses, almost all PD patients will experience constipation, sometimes in very impactful ways. Patients can end up hospitalized to treat bowel obstruction. To avoid complications of constipation, it's important to really tailor a patient's bowel regimen as an outpatient and to maintain it during a hospitalization. Ask patients and caregivers about the usual bowel regimen on admission.

Prevention is the best approach. Above all, maintain good hydration and the patient's usual diet. If the patient regularly uses stool softeners or MiraLAX, make sure this continues on schedule. Milk of magnesia, suppositories, enemas, and laxatives that speed up transit such as lactulose, can be safely used. Using opiates can exacerbate constipation. Patients with PD on opiates should be monitored more closely for GI disturbances.

SENSORY ISSUES

Sensory issues are an underappreciated aspect of PD. Loss of smell (anosmia) can be a symptom early on, even before the PD diagnosis is made. Later on, loss of taste (hypogeusia) may occur.

Losing the senses of smell and taste makes food much less appealing. Adding a lot of salt or sugar can help a little by making the food have some flavor. Adding more flavorful foods and spices that wake up the taste buds can help. Parkinson's patients should aim for a brain-healthy diet that is high in green leafy vegetables, fresh fruit, whole grains, and healthy fats. In the hospital, rehab, or nursing home setting, with uninspired choices for the food tray, not much may be able to be done to liven up the diet.

SWALLOWING PROBLEMS (DYSPHAGIA)

Dysphagia is a common problem for PD patients. The best treatment is good, dedicated speech therapy with a swallowing specialist. Hospitalized patients should have a quick swallow evaluation by a nurse or speech therapist when they're admitted. Ask the patient and their care-givers about what they usually eat at home to determine how limiting the dysphagia is.

Hospital staff should be aware of the risk of choking and aspiration for these patients. Patients can avoid or reduce choking by using chin tucks, postural changes, or whatever other maneuvers the patient usually uses or the swallowing specialist has recommended. Timing of PD medications is critical, as delayed dosing of PD meds can exacerbate dysphagia.

Every patient will be different and some will need dietary modifications. Foods may need to be pureed or ground;

liquids may need to be thickened. These modifications aren't very appetizing, so patients must be monitored for adequate food intake and dehydration. Consult with the hospital dietitian to find ways to make the food as appetizing as possible.

NUTRITIONAL ISSUES

In some cases, a dietary interaction can occur between protein and levodopa. Meals with protein should be separated from medication doses. If the patient takes levodopa too close to a meal high in protein (a portion larger than the size of the patient's fist), the protein blocks the levodopa from being absorbed, and the dose will not be as effective. Meal orders should be reviewed to be sure protein isn't excessive. Some protein is fine, but triple cheeseburgers are out.

Protein-levodopa competition can cause issues with off times. Meal trays should be timed to the dosing schedule. Ideally, levodopa should be taken 30 to 60 minutes before a meal to allow the drug to be absorbed quickly, before food can interfere. This is true of controlled-release versions as well. These versions take longer to kick in, and if they're taken with a meal, they'll sit in the stomach instead of starting to work.

Maintaining good nutritional status is very important.

Consult the hospital nutritionist with any dietary concerns for PD patients.

DROOLING

Drooling is a common symptom of PD; patients may choke on their saliva. Drooling isn't caused by overproduction of saliva; rather, it's because people with PD can't clear secretions effectively. Small sips of water every hour or so can help engage the clearing reflex. Swallowing problems and drooling can get worse during off periods and can be worsened by delay in the medications. The dopamine dose may need to be increased. If the drooling is very bothersome, anticholinergic drugs that dry the mouth, such as glycopyrrolate (Robinul), can be given.

Drooling can be distressing for patients because it's so socially embarrassing. We have patients who stop socializing because they're so aware of their drooling. Speech and swallowing therapy can help quite a bit with drooling. The Lee Silverman program (see below) is specifically designed to improve this symptom and other speech-related problems. If the hospital offers this form of therapy, it should be considered. Otherwise, order standard speech therapy.

LEE SILVERMAN VOICE TREATMENT

The Lee Silverman Voice Treatment (LSVT) is a specialized and very helpful form of speech therapy developed just for people with PD. LSVT LOUD was developed in 1987. It can really improve speech and related issues, including disorders of articulation, diminished facial expression, and impaired swallowing. It improves vocal loudness through exercises that stimulate the muscles of the voice box and speech mechanisms to maximize speech intelligibility. LSVT can make a substantial difference in the patient's quality of life and ability to communicate. The program is taught to the patient by a specially trained speech therapist in 16 sessions over the course of a month (four individual training sessions of one hour each per week).

The same principles of LSVT LOUD have started to be applied to limb movement in people with PD in a program called LSVT BIG. The program trains patients to increase the amplitude of their limb and body movements. The program can be very helpful for improving gait, posture, balance, and the ability to perform activities of daily living. The program is taught to the patient by a specially trained physical or occupational therapist in 16 sessions over the course of a month (four individual training sessions of one hour each per week).

For both LOUD and BIG therapy, the patient is given

exercises to do between sessions and to maintain gains after therapy ends. Doing the exercises is key to success, so inpatients should be encouraged to practice. If the hospital has LSVT BIG- and LOUD-certified therapists, consider a consultation for PD patients.

To find certified LSVT LOUD and BIG therapists, check the website at www.lsvtglobal.com.

PAIN

Pain and paresthesias may be symptoms of Parkinson's, especially if they worsen in the off state. This type of pain isn't the same as neuropathy. It may be a perceived sensation. In these patients, treatment of PD may help the sensation of pain; delay or omission of PD meds may exacerbate these symptoms.

PD can be the etiology of pain and can also exacerbate pain. Patients with PD may experience different types of PD pain, such as pain in muscles and joints, pain in internal organs such as the bowel or the bladder, fluctuating pains, pain at night, or headaches. They can also experience other pain unrelated to PD, such as radicular pains or knee or hip pain. Often, these pains will also fluctuate with Parkinson's symptoms.

Muscle and joint pains can be treated with anti-inflammatories and also with physical therapy, particularly if the pain is in the back, shoulder, or knee. PD medications can also be helpful. Cramping pains in the abdomen can be quite distressing and fluctuate with on and off cycles. These may respond to PD medications or muscle relaxants. Opiates may exacerbate this type of pain by causing constipation; ensuring constipation is addressed may also help. Parkinson's disease can cause motor fluctuations that appear as involuntary dystonia caused by rigid posturing of the muscles or extremities and cramping of the calf or leg muscles. Massage and stretching may help. These pains often emerge in off periods, so it is critical to maintain strict adherence to the PD medication regimen.

Patients with PD may also experience pain or unpleasant sensations during sleep or as they are trying to go to sleep. Restless leg symptoms can affect these patients. Maintaining a reasonable sleep environment in the hospital may help, as may PD medications such as dopamine agonists.

We again return to the central theme of this book: adherence to the customized medication regimen of PD patients (often painstakingly fine-tuned in the office) when these patients are admitted to the hospital is essential.

Standard non-opiate pain medications are generally safe

for PD patients, although some interactions may occur with tramadol (Ultram) and MAO-B inhibitors. Opiates can be administered, with the understanding of potential deleterious effects of confusion and constipation. Meperidine (Demerol) should not be given to those on MAO-B inhibitors such as selegiline. In general, we try to avoid meperidine altogether.

FALLS AND FALL PREVENTION

Falls are a leading cause of hospitalization and rehospitalization for PD patients. Fall prevention is crucial. This should include a home safety evaluation before discharge to ensure that the environment is open and safe and that patients have adequate tools for safe mobility, including walkers, canes, walking sticks, or even a wheelchair if necessary.

A physical therapist should perform a fall assessment for all inpatients with PD. If the patient is a fall risk—and all will likely be—the usual fall prevention precautions must be taken. When helping patients with getting in and out of bed, using the bathroom, and so on, be alert to fall risk, just as you would be for any other patient.

During the inpatient stay, balance training with a physical therapist can be helpful. This is particularly important in the rehab setting.

After discharge from the hospital or rehab, services should be established to help prevent falls at home through a home safety check and home physical therapy. Stairs, for instance, can be difficult for PD patients. Their balance is impaired, and often their depth perception may be affected as well. They might mistake the riser height, thinking the step is higher or lower than it actually is. They need to be taught how to be cautious on stairs.

Once again, we emphasize the importance of maintaining adherence to the patient's PD medication regimen. Ample evidence demonstrates higher risk of falls in the hospital if PD patients do not receive their medications on time.

THE MULTIDISCIPLINARY TEAM

The multidisciplinary team approach is key to providing comprehensive care for every PD patient. The team approach ensures that all the patient's providers are in communication with each other and with the patient and caregivers. Each specialist has their own area of expertise for Parkinson's symptoms, but the patient's care must be holistic and coordinated with all the other specialists.

The team includes physicians and other healthcare practitioners, such as physical therapists, occupational and speech therapists, and especially family members and other caregivers. In addition, the team is enhanced by the availability of social workers, local support group members, and patient advocates.

In our experience, the PD multidisciplinary team works best when the patient's neurologist (preferably a movement disorders specialist) is the team coordinator, like the captain of the ship. The neurologist should be the point person in coordinating the team's approach and care. The primary care physician should manage the regular care and ensure that non-PD issues are treated. Along with managing comorbidities, the primary care doctor should maintain contact with the team. Test results should be reported to the team. If a patient is hospitalized, notes are critical for knowing if the issues have been reported and discussed earlier.

Nurses, nursing assistants, physical therapists, occupational therapists, speech therapists, social workers, and everyone else should always advocate for these patients. If they notice something about a hospitalized PD patient, they should be encouraged to say something, and the information should be shared with the team.

THE ROLE OF THERAPISTS

Medications can help many of the symptoms of PD. They are complemented by nonpharmacological modalities that help in areas where medications may not. Gait, balance, speech, and swallowing can be helped with exercise and with therapy. Physical, occupational, and speech therapists play an important role in the care of these patients, both inside and outside of the hospital.

Therapists play a huge role in treating these patients. Patients should do physical therapy, occupational therapy, and speech therapy in the hospital, but they also need these services regularly as outpatients. The care team should be as proactive as possible in helping patients get these therapies on a regular basis.

Patients rely on and utilize these resources so much so that they may use up their annual health insurance benefits for services such as physical therapy before the year is finished. For these patients, we recommend transitioning to a wellness program or a community-based exercise class. These may have some costs, but many programs for older adults are low-cost or free. Social workers can help patients find programs as part of discharge planning. Patients can also check with their state office for the aging to find local programs, and with the Parkinson's Foundation. We have patients who spread their benefits out over the year, arranging some sessions, taking a break but continuing to practice their therapy and exercise, and then resuming.

PSYCHOLOGY AND PSYCHIATRY

Patients with Parkinson's can be prone to depression, apathy, anxiety, cognitive decline, and other mental health issues. It's important to remember that these are nonmotor symptoms of the disease, caused by changes in brain chemistry. They are as much biological as psychological. Psychotherapy is helpful, but the therapist needs to be aware of the brain changes that underlie the mental health issues. Drug treatment with antianxiety and antidepressant drugs may be needed. Drugs must be carefully prescribed and monitored; consulting with the neurologist and primary care physician is recommended.

ADVOCATES

Community advocates are an excellent source of practical information about local services. These people exist to help. Encourage patients and their families to use them. Support groups can be really helpful for positivity and sharing experiences. They're sometimes more valuable for the caregivers than the patients.

FAMILY AND LOVED ONES

The importance of family, loved ones, and caregivers is often underestimated and underrecognized. These people are very dedicated and make a huge difference in how well a patient does. Selfless as they are, they are also subject to exhaustion, depression, and burnout. We counsel caregivers to leave time for themselves and, specifically, to avoid becoming socially isolated.

Parkinson's is primarily a disease of older adults, which means spouses who are caretakers may well have their own medical issues (and sometimes patients with PD are also caregivers). We counsel caregivers to be mindful of their own medical needs. Be proactive and ask the caregiver, "How are you doing?" Often, patients end up in a nursing home or hospice because their caregivers can't handle the responsibility anymore. They may not be physically capable of it, and they may also lack support or adequate resources. Caregiver burnout is a genuine problem, so don't overlook them. They truly are the patients' best advocates. In an important way, the patient is only doing as well as their caregiver.

BRINGING IT ALL TOGETHER: COMMUNICATION

Communication, communication, communication. It's just as important as continuity of care.

Lack of communication is poor communication. We see this all too often. If the people caring for someone with PD don't communicate, then they're not advocating for the patient. Team members are often overworked; hospitals and facilities are often understaffed. Spending extra time to work out an issue with a Parkinson's patient may seem like a luxury, but it can make a huge difference. Taking a little extra time now can save a lot of time later by keeping a small problem from turning into a big one. Sometimes all it takes is a quick phone call to the neurologist to close the loop.

SYMPTOMS AND TREATMENTS

SYMPTOM	TREATMENT
Apathy	Levodopa Psychiatric consult
Anxiety	Benzodiazepine
Constipation	Diet/hydration MiraLAX Other over-the-counter products
Delirium	Reassurance Check for underlying cause (e.g., infection)
Drooling	Speech therapy/LSVT therapy Anticholinergic drugs
Hallucinations	Insight retained: reassurance Insight lost: reassurance, quetiapine (Seroquel)
Neurogenic orthostatic hypotension	Elevate bed head Fall precautions Drugs: fludrocortisone (Florinef), midodrine (Amatine, ProAmatine), droxidopa (Northera)
Loss of smell/taste	Nutrition consult
Pain and paresthesias	Standard drugs; avoid narcotics Avoid meperidine (Demerol) with selegiline
Sleep disorders	Sleep hygiene Evening dopamine Benzodiazepine (Klonopin)

PART III

—

ADMISSION: PROBLEMS AND SOLUTIONS

CHAPTER 6

The Incomplete Assessment

Patients with Parkinson's disease who happen to be admitted to the hospital have a higher chance of developing complications from their hospitalization. In addition to whatever health issue has brought them to the hospital, these patients face additional risks related to incomplete assessment, medication and timing issues, and perioperative issues. All staff members should always bear the patient's PD status in mind. Incomplete assessment of their symptoms, history, and medication regimen; delays or omissions or substitution of PD medications; and administration of contraindicated medications compound their risks. Patients with PD not only have a higher chance of getting admitted to the hospital for non-Parkinson's issues but also have a higher chance of developing complications in the hospital such as falls, dysphagia, and confusion. Ample evidence suggests missing doses of medication or delays of administering these medications significantly increases these risks.

Problems for a hospitalized PD patient often start with admission to the hospital and compound from there. A major problem on admission is incomplete assessment.

A thorough assessment is crucial whenever a PD patient needs to be hospitalized, on an emergency or planned basis. The assessment should include a very close look at the patient's history, with particular attention to the medications and dosing schedule.

The goal of the assessment is to determine the correct medications and schedule, minimize medication errors, and avoid problems down the road.

GLORIA AND GEORGE: TWO PATIENTS

The cases of Gloria and George are both examples of how incomplete assessment can lead to a cascade of complications over the course of a hospitalization. They are based on real experiences we have had when PD patients are admitted to the hospital. Elements from these stories occur across the country whenever a PD patient is admitted to the hospital.

GLORIA: A VISIT THROUGH THE EMERGENCY ROOM

Gloria is a 73-year-old female who has had Parkinson's for about 10 years. She and her elderly husband come to the emergency room one evening because Gloria is in respiratory distress. They have forgotten to bring her medications list or medications.

Gloria is having shortness of breath, and it is difficult to obtain a history from her. Her husband, who is the primary caregiver, tells the staff that Gloria has PD and takes levodopa six times a day. He is uncertain about the exact dose but knows the times and knows that she has missed her usual evening dose.

The presence of Gloria's PD takes a back seat for the ED staff. Their exam and attention is centered on her breathing difficulty. The missed dose doesn't seem that important, and her caregiver isn't consulted about it any further. Gloria is admitted to the hospital with pneumonia.

Gloria spends many hours in the emergency room, and by the time she is sent up to the medical floor, she is experiencing motor symptoms and is very confused. Her caregiver, by this point overwhelmed and exhausted, is very concerned about her breathing. He tells the new nursing staff about the PD medications and that she has missed some doses. The nurses assure Gloria's husband that they will make sure the orders are placed. At that moment, however, their main concern is her respiratory status and the orders aren't placed right away. Gloria is now on supplemental oxygen and is getting some breathing treatments.

Because her oxygenation doesn't improve, Gloria is now placed in the ICU. The doctors and nurses finally get her back on her usual PD medication, but Gloria doesn't do well in the ICU. The noise, constant light, lack of sleep, and hypoxia make her confusion worse, and she starts to have hallucinations. Gloria is given the antipsychotic drug haloperidol (Haldol). This drug is commonly used in the ICU, but it is contraindicated in PD. By the time the error is noticed, Gloria is much worse. She requires intubation as her motor symptoms worsen and her respiratory efforts diminish. Ultimately, her confusion and poor respiratory efforts make it very difficult to wean her off the ventilator.

After a very challenging hospitalization, Gloria is finally ready for discharge. She has been deconditioned, is not capable of performing any of her activities of daily living, and is now too much for her husband to care for. He can no longer provide the level of care she now needs, so Gloria ends up in a nursing home, where she may have to spend the rest of her life.

What Went Wrong?

Gloria ended up in the nursing home because of several potentially preventable errors.

The problems begin with Gloria's lack of an accurate, up-to-date medications list. In the confusion of an emergency situation, patients and caretakers often forget the list or realize it hasn't been kept current. Without the list, the emergency room staff should have spent more time with both Gloria and her husband to get as accurate an idea as possible of her current medications and symptoms. Alternatively, they should have reached out to her neurologist. Because they didn't have a list of her medications to remind them, and because they were focused on Gloria's respiratory distress, her PD status was pushed to the background. The staff should have been more aware of it and should have asked her husband for the names of Gloria's PD doctor and primary care doctor. The staff should have contacted them as soon as possible. They would have been very helpful for coordinating her emergency room care.

Once Gloria arrived on the medical floor, her PD status was still not brought forward enough for immediate action on her missed medications. A neurology consult should have been ordered. The neurologist could have educated the staff about the importance of timely medication and how to deal with psychosis and cognitive impairment in

PD patients. The serious error of giving Gloria a contra-indicated drug for her hallucinations should never have occurred. People with PD have a reduction in their brain supply of neurotransmitters, in particular dopamine. The Parkinson's medications are aimed at replenishing the dopamine or mimicking the effects in some fashion. Anti-psychotic medications block dopamine and can cause significant worsening of PD symptoms for that reason.

Managing PD patients in the ICU is also challenging, especially if the patients are intubated for ventilatory support. Most PD meds are oral, and delivering the medications when patients do not have an orogastric or nasogastric tube is not possible. These patients are at even higher risk of deterioration as their ability to expand their chest is diminished if they are not getting the PD meds. Trying to wean them off the ventilator then becomes more and more difficult with this vicious circle.

GEORGE: COMING IN FOR AN ELECTIVE SURGERY

George is in his sixties and has had PD for several years. He's otherwise fairly healthy and has come to the hospital for elective knee replacement surgery. He's accompanied by his son. During his pre-op admission, he presents a medications list and tells the staff that he takes carbi-dopa/levodopa (Sinemet) four times a day at 6:00 a.m.,

10:00 a.m., 2:00 p.m., and 6:00 p.m., and also takes the dopamine agonist ropinirole (Requip) with each dose.

In preparation for the surgery, George was told not to take anything by mouth starting at midnight the night before. When he arrives at the hospital that morning, he has already missed his first morning dose; he misses the second while waiting in the pre-op area.

George's surgery starts at noon and is completed successfully, with no complications. By 2:00 p.m., he's in the recovery room and appears alert. He is due for his third dose of Sinemet, but this is withheld for fear of aspiration, as his diet also has not been ordered.

Earlier, when the orthopedic surgery physician assistant (PA) put in orders for Sinemet four times a day, the electronic medical record (EMR) defaulted to a standard dosing schedule instead of George's individualized schedule. The PA didn't notice. At the same time, the EMR alerted the PA that Requip wasn't in the hospital formulary and suggested bromocriptine instead. The PA accepted the suggestion.

At 4:00 p.m., the physical therapists come to see George. By this time, George has missed his third carbidopa/levodopa dose of the day and hasn't received ropinirole either. His knee is immobilized, but he's supposed to be immobile for one day, so the physical therapists think this is normal. They help him stand and move a bit but leave the knee exercises for the following day. George is stiff and unable to move because he hasn't had his PD meds, but the hospital staff doesn't realize it. George finally gets some levodopa that evening at 8:00 p.m. By then, he is very immobile.

The next morning, George gets his meds later than usual; the substitution of bromocriptine for Requip makes him very drowsy. At this point, George is so immobile that when the physical therapists arrive, he can't even get out of bed. He complains of being stiff, in spasm, and in pain. The nurse examines him, notices rigidity, and assumes that it is because of pain. George is on pain medication, but even after it is given, he remains immobile—and he's miserable.

The staff is starting to realize that a medication problem is behind George's immobility, but still, another hour passes before he receives his usual dose. Because his medication schedule has been so thrown off, however, he remains very immobile. He can't do physical therapy. Instead of being able to go home shortly after the surgery as planned, George ends up staying in the hospital for two weeks. From there, instead of going home and resuming a fairly independent life, George gets sent to a rehab facility.

What Went Wrong?

The root cause of the problem was the surgeon's assumption that George's surgery would be like anyone else's. This is never the case for people with PD. George's routine surgery turned into a disaster for reasons all related to his medication.

The cascade of problems started that morning, even before George arrived at the hospital. He was told by the surgeon's nurse not to take his medications before the surgery, missing a dose of the PD meds even before arriving to the hospital. Then he was NPO (nothing by mouth) in the pre-op area and missed another dose. Even worse, his next dose wasn't given in post-op after he woke up. Then his evening dose was administered much later than usual.

There is no reason for PD patients to skip their drugs prior to surgery. These patients should *never* skip their medications, even if they are awaiting surgery or are NPO for some other reason. The importance of the medication far outweighs any risk. George was awake enough to take his usual afternoon dose, but this was never administered.

PD medications should be resumed as soon as possible after surgery. To avoid missed doses, people with PD should be scheduled for surgery as early in the morning as possible. If that's not possible, every effort should be made to give their medication in the holding area as scheduled until they go into surgery.

George's individualized dosing schedule was inadvertently changed when the PA automatically accepted the standard four-times-a-day schedule from the EMR. The problem was compounded by the erroneous substitution of bromocriptine for Requip. Even though both of these medications are in the same class, substitution of medications for PD patients is not appropriate and it can result in lack of efficacy, or side effects.

All the medication errors were avoidable. In particular, the incorrect dosing and drug substitution should never have happened. The surgeon should have included a note about the individualized dosing schedule in George's chart. Even without the note, the PA should have been aware of the crucial importance of dose timing for PD patients and should have overridden the EMR default schedule with the individual customized schedule. The PA should also not have automatically accepted the substitution of bromocriptine for Requip. The drug regimen of PD patients is carefully worked out and should not be changed. Instead of accepting the drug substitution, the PA should have checked with George and his caregivers to see if they brought his Requip from home. Hospital regulations generally allow patients to take medications from home if they are in the original container and are given to the nurses to dispense.

As this drug disaster unfolded, George's son told the nurse he thought his father needed his medication. Because George was still fairly independent and his son wasn't that familiar with his condition, he didn't press the issue. Besides, the surgical post-op area was even busier than usual that afternoon and evening, and the nurses simply didn't pay enough attention. They never asked him if he had brought his father's Requip from home, even though he had.

When George was in recovery, the physical therapists mistook his PD immobility for the lingering effects of the anesthesia. They left, thinking he simply wasn't ready, instead of realizing that he was frozen because he needed his meds. Had they spoken with the nurse, they might have realized the problem and known that once George took his medication, he would soon be mobile enough for therapy. Instead, they walked away.

From Bad to Worse

At the rehab center, the cycle repeats itself: George's medicines aren't appropriately ordered and administered. On his second day in the rehab hospital, George develops significant leg swelling. An ultrasound of his leg reveals a large deep vein thrombosis. The immobility has taken its toll. The rehab hospital sends him back to the hospital.

Back in the hospital, George is started on warfarin (Coumadin). The hospitalization has set George back, however, and his medications need to be adjusted. While the hospital struggles to determine the right doses, George is still unable to mobilize effectively. He gets sent back to the rehab center, but his poor balance and lack of mobility make him a fall risk. The physical therapists working with George are inexperienced with PD and don't realize how poor his balance is. George falls during physical therapy. Because he's on warfarin, he develops a large hematoma around the knee. After a few days, the swelling is so severe that he gets sent back to the hospital again. His knee is infected, and the surgeon has to remove his knee replacement.

The fall during physical therapy could have been avoided if the therapists had had more experience working with PD patients. They could have been educated about the immobility, balance, and posture problems these patients have, but they weren't.

The routine knee replacement that was supposed to help George retain his mobility and independence has turned into a disaster. His PD symptoms have gotten much worse, and he's disabled by the knee surgery. He can barely move, but his lack of physical activity only makes the PD worse. This time, George goes from the hospital to a nursing home. In the space of a month, he has gone from being mobile and mostly independent to being wheelchair-bound in a nursing home.

ALTERNATIVE SCENARIOS

In both the above scenarios, from the first interaction with the patients, the hospital staff failed to appropriately assess the patients and to correctly identify medications and dosing times. The staff failed to appreciate the urgency of learning which medications these patients were on, didn't understand why substitutions should not have been made, and were unaware of the urgency of dose timing.

Parkinson's medications must be given on time!

Even in a crowded emergency room or busy hospital floor, the extra effort must be made. Patients who don't get the right drugs at the right time are very likely to end up with an extended hospital stay and potential complications that leave them worse off than before.

For both Gloria and George, the hospital staff missed multiple opportunities for effective intervention. They could have gotten a better understanding of the correct dosing simply by taking the time to talk with the patients and their caregivers. In fact, they could have intervened simply by noting the medication times and working to find a way to get the patient a medication that was not on the formulary.

While in our busy routines in the hospital, it seems at best impractical and at worst impossible to take even the few minutes to make the extra effort for a PD patient. Making the extra calls, asking the extra questions, or spending more time wrestling with the EMRs to add the timing of medications and override standard default timing suggestions can seem too difficult. Even so, it is imperative to do so. Anything less can put the patient in harm's way.

CHAPTER 7

Medication Timing and Contraindications

Problems with medications are widespread at healthcare facilities, including hospitals, rehab centers, and nursing homes.

Many people with Parkinson's disease (PD) require significantly high doses of medication and significantly high frequency of medications. They live dose to dose; their ability to move depends on whether the medication is in their system and working. Their ability to move and function over time decreases as the disease progresses. By adjusting the mix of medications and their timing, we can do a lot to manage the symptoms and help the patient stay as independent as possible for as long as possible.

FINE-TUNING THE DRUG REGIMEN

When a Parkinson's patient progresses to a more disabling stage of the disease, the neurologist, the patient, and family members discuss medications in significant detail. The drug regimen that works best for the patient often becomes increasingly complex, with more frequent doses on a more complicated schedule, and with additional drugs added to the mix. Drug side effects can become more severe and distressing.

The only way to know if the changes in the drug regimen are working is for the patient to try them. The neurologist writes out the schedule, the patient goes home and tries it. The patient or caregiver keeps a symptom diary and then returns at a later visit with feedback. Perhaps the regimen worked well in the morning but not in the afternoon. Or maybe the side effects of the larger dose were too annoying, or the new drug caused nausea.

The team makes adjustments. Now, perhaps, the patient is supposed to take the medication before meals, or after meals, or take a drug every other day. Getting the patient onto an effective drug regimen is a highly customized and laborious process that involves the whole treatment team. To develop the best regimen possible under the circumstances takes a lot of work and a bit of luck.

All the work of getting a patient onto a drug regimen

that's working well can be thrown completely off by a hospitalization. In the hospital, these very fragile patients are at the mercy of a chaotic environment where the medication subtleties can be overlooked, especially by healthcare providers who are unfamiliar with PD. This lack of understanding is unfortunately common.

In our experience, most clinicians aren't aware of the importance of the timing of these medications or the risks of contraindicated medications. The same is true of the nursing staff. These deficiencies in knowledge lead to medication delays, inappropriate drug substitutions, and avoidable drug interactions.

Some literature indicates that people with PD end up being admitted to the hospital 50 percent more often than those without Parkinson's. Most of the time, the admission is not for PD but for common conditions that bring most people to the hospital—not only emergencies such as heart attacks and broken hips but also for elective surgery. They also happen to have PD.

The number of patients with PD who enter the hospital over the course of a year isn't very high. The small population means that the hospital staff has limited experience with these patients. Educating them about the best approaches may be a challenge because of the small numbers, but it is still imperative.

BYPASSING THE HOSPITAL ROUTINE

In the hospital setting, prescribing and administering medication can be inflexible. When a medication is prescribed for three times a day, it's routinely given at default intervals. Similarly, the default for four times a day is six hours apart. The electronic medical record (EMR) will often determine the dosing schedules, and the ordering doctor simply clicks to agree to it. We may do this because it is easier or because we may not be aware of the importance of timing of medications, but it's also because trying to bypass the EMR defaults is difficult. It requires a lot of time-consuming extra clicks; sometimes it's actually impossible. The extra steps to change the times can be so frustrating that the ordering practitioners simply don't take them.

On the hospital floor, the nurses may be busy with several patients. They know that getting patients their meds on schedule is important, but if the timing is missed, they may feel it's not the end of the world. A patient with high blood pressure who is supposed to take their medicine at 9:00 a.m. will be OK if it's given at 11:00 a.m. instead. Most patients have manageable conditions that aren't very dependent on the timing of their drugs, but this doesn't translate well to Parkinson's medications.

In the busy hospital environment, the static defaults forced by the EMR are easy to accept—they make sense for most patients and cut back on medication errors. But when very fragile Parkinson's patients are in the hospital, simple EMR medication schedules can't accommodate the highly detailed instructions for their medications. The medication program doesn't get followed. When we place these patients in the hospital, they're suddenly at the mercy of the frenetic hospital environment. This is when problems occur.

Most PD patients who come to the hospital end up with disrupted medication regimens. This has been demonstrated in numerous journal articles. Seventy-five percent of PD patients in the hospital don't get their medications correctly. They receive the wrong doses, the wrong timing, or the wrong medication. About 60 percent will have serious complications as a result.

For some patients with Parkinson's, missing their medication by even 15 minutes can have significant deleterious effects. It can result in dysphagia, which only makes the medication problem even worse. It can also cause confusion or falls in the hospital. Notably, it can increase the length of stay. Parkinson's patients often have their hospitalizations extended beyond what would be expected for their admitting diagnosis.

IMPROVING EDUCATION

The lack of education about Parkinson's disease and best

practices for hospitalized patients is a major but generally overlooked reason for the problems these patients encounter. Within the Parkinson's community, we are seeing a movement to educate practitioners, patients, and hospitals. The Parkinson's Foundation has developed an educational program that emphasizes the importance of giving medications on time, every time.

In the United States, hospital regulations may be obstacles to giving timely medication. Hospitals are required by their regulatory bodies to have very strict rules about patients bringing their own medicine to the hospital. For PD patients, these rules can end up being harmful, especially in emergency situations, where the busy emergency room staff can't provide drugs according to the patient's individual schedule, and where hospital formularies don't include a drug the patient needs.

While most hospitals have provisions for medications not in the hospital formulary and brought in by the patients, the staff may not be familiar with them. They need education about the process and advocates who can ensure this process is taking place when needed.

WHAT'S THE SCHEDULE?

When someone with PD is admitted to the hospital, flags should go up that this patient has Parkinson's and needs medicine on time. Sticking to the medication schedule should become a standard of care for these patients, just as managing diabetes and heart attacks have well-known automatic protocols.

Identifying patients with Parkinson's is a crucial first step. In our hospital, PD patients are flagged electronically with a pop-up banner every time the chart is opened. We also will be utilizing a wristband on the patient that identifies them as Parkinson's patients. This goes well beyond the simple fall-risk wristband. Bear in mind that while we take the fall-risk wristband for granted today, it was once an innovative idea. We feel the PD wristband is something that should become standard practice. It identifies the patient not just as a fall risk but also reminds the staff that this patient needs special medication management.

Even when the doctors and nurses are aware of the importance of sticking to the drug schedule for a Parkinson's patient, they may not know what the schedule is. Communicating with the patient, caregiver, and the outpatient medical team is key. The patient may not have brought a medications list to the hospital, or it may not be up to date. We often fine-tune the patient's medication schedule. If the patient calls and says they're feeling very stiff, for instance, we might say to add an extra dose of levodopa at noon, but that information might not make it to the list the patient brings to the hospital. Get the information from the patient and caregiver. Check with the patient's neurologist or primary care physician if there is any doubt at all about the drugs, doses, and schedule.

The patient and caregiver should be specifically asked about what medications they take, the dose of these medications, and the exact time they are taken. The answers should be as precise as possible. If the patient takes a drug at exactly 6:15 p.m., that should be documented. How long the drug takes to work and how long it lasts varies considerably from patient to patient. What the patient needs and when should take precedence over the EMR-generated medication schedule.

Medications for patients with PD cannot be replaced or substituted. The drug the patient takes is exactly what needs to be given. If the drug isn't in the hospital formulary, an alternative *should not* be substituted. For blood pressure drugs, one beta-blocker can be substituted for another, usually without any real issues. Similarly, one statin drug is generally more or less interchangeable with another. Parkinson's medications are different. Not only are PD patients very dependent on the timing of a drug, but they're also very dependent on the formulation. Even variations in the same drug's formulation, such as an extended-release form, can change how effective it is for the individual patient.

Nurses caring for Parkinson's patients should ask if they

have their own medicine if it's not in the hospital formulary. Our instructions for patients having elective surgery include telling them to bring their medicines, in the original bottle, to the hospital. That should be the standard for any Parkinson's patients in the hospital. Some physicians may not know it, but this is a perfectly appropriate practice. Usually the pharmacy will need to verify the medication and the nurses will have to administer the drug.

Not all hospitals carry as wide a range of drugs as are needed for PD patients. This unfortunate situation ultimately comes down to economics. There simply aren't enough hospitalized Parkinson's patients over the course of a year to make stocking all PD medications economically viable. Indeed, when hospitals are able to see the importance of this process, they become stakeholders and partners in the elevation of the care for these patients. We are fortunate that our hospital is such an organization.

Nurses should also make sure that PD patients are not told to skip their medicine when they are NPO (nothing by mouth). They should always be given their medicines with a small sip of water or crushed in applesauce if necessary. Even if the patient is being prepped for surgery, the Parkinson's meds should be given on schedule. The idea of NPO before surgery is with regard to food and should not apply to medications—and in particular not to Parkinson's patients taking their PD medications.

PATIENT INITIATIVE

Patients and their caregivers should keep a detailed, up-to-date list of all medications, doses, and timing. They should always bring it with them to the hospital. In the stress of an emergency hospitalization, the list may be forgotten. We suggest to patients that they make multiple copies of the list and keep them in various places, such as wallets, handbags, and overnight bags that will probably go with them to the hospital. In addition, we suggest giving the list to all caregivers, family members, and loved ones so that someone else is likely to have it when it's needed. Patients should also have contact information for their neurologist and primary care physician and a trusted caregiver with them when they arrive at the hospital. To be sure that information is readily available, we suggest including it on the medications list, along with emergency contact information.

Patients and caregivers often don't understand the complex mechanics of a hospitalization. They may not understand who does what in the emergency room and on the floor. They may not grasp the procedures that control how orders are put in and medications are given. Those orders, administered by the physician, are very specific—they can't be changed unless a doctor says so. An error in medication that creeps in at the start of the hospitalization may take persistence on the part of the patient and caregiver to correct.

When patients and caregivers go to the hospital, they have to be advocates for themselves. Certain errors of hospitalization can be only avoided by ensuring that patients explain exactly which medications they take and exactly what time. The explanations may need to be given multiple times to different staff members. Patients and caregivers can't assume that telling one staff member about medications one time is enough to make sure the information is communicated. They need to remind everyone they encounter about their PD and their meds.

Even if a patient has been at the hospital before or is part of a medical practice associated with the hospital, their records won't necessarily be available. Unless the patient or caregiver tells the physician or nurse about all their medicines and how they are taken, there's no good way for the hospital to have this information. Often, we hear patients say, "Well, it's in the records." But it's not. We can't rely on records or a doctor's verbal instructions. We also can't be sure that the patient's medications list gets accurately transcribed into the EMR. Patients and caregivers need to speak up if they see that errors have been made.

CONTRAINDICATED MEDICATIONS

Several commonly used medications can affect Parkinson's patients quite significantly. Unfortunately, many of these medications are used frequently in the hospital either as routine medications after surgery or for control of pain, or are some common medications that are used to address a confused or agitated patient.

Knowledge about these potentially harmful medications is quite important to keep Parkinson's patients safe in the hospital.

NAUSEA MEDICATION

Metoclopramide (Reglan) and prochlorperazine (Compazine) are commonly used post-surgery and after anesthesia to help reduce nausea. These medications are dopamine antagonists and can affect patients with Parkinson's by worsening their symptoms. In lieu of these medicines, ondansetron (Zofran) and trimethobenzamide (Tigan), which are safer in the Parkinson's population, can be used. Because of the large use of anti-nausea medication in the hospital, we find this class of medications to be the largest offenders in PD patients. A serious effort has to be directed at addressing these medications.

ANTIPSYCHOTIC MEDICATION

In general, most atypical and typical antipsychotics are contraindicated in Parkinson's patients because of their antidopaminergic effects. Medications such as haloperidol (Haldol), chlorpromazine (Thorazine), risperidone (Risperdal), and olanzapine (Zyprexa) should be avoided. Safer medications are quetiapine (Seroquel), clozapine (Clozaril), or pimavanserin (Nuplazid).

ANTIDEPRESSANTS

Tricyclic antidepressants such as amitriptyline and nortriptyline should be avoided with PD. Safer medications are escitalopram (Lexapro), venlafaxine (Effexor), fluoxetine (Prozac), sertraline (Zoloft), paroxetine (Paxil), and citalopram (Celexa).

OTHER MEDICATIONS

Isoniazid (Nydrazid), phenytoin (Dilantin), and papaverine (Pavabid, Papacon, Pavagen, Pavacot) should be avoided. In addition, if any patient is taking an MAO-B inhibitor such as rasagiline or selegiline, meperidine, tramadol, and droperidol should be avoided.

AWARE IN CARE

The Parkinson's Foundation has created a very valuable

program called Aware in Care that is designed to help people with Parkinson's get the best care possible during a hospital stay. The program has created a free patient safety kit for patients facing hospitalization. The kit contains a very useful medication form where the patient can record all medications, the dosages, the timing, the condition the drugs treat, and when the patient started taking them. The form also has space to list other conditions, doctors, and care partners. All this information is critical to have in place before the patient is inundated by the chaos and disruptions of hospitalization.

The Aware in Care kit also provides a medical alert wallet card, action plans to help patients prepare for both emergency and elective hospitalizations, a stack of preprinted reminder slips about PD that patients can hand to anyone they encounter, and some background information about PD that can be useful for educating hospital staff, including a list of contraindicated medications and alternatives.

We support this program and will be providing our patients the Aware in Care kit. We recommend that they fill out the medication form and pack it in the kit along with a 48-hour supply of their medications.

For more information or to request a free kit, contact the Parkinson's Foundation at www.awareincare.org or call 1-800-4PD-INFO (473-4636). The Parkinson's Foundation, formed by the merger of the National Parkinson Foundation and the Parkinson's Disease Foundation, provides education and resources for patients, caregivers, and medical professionals. It is an excellent source of accurate, up-to-date information for patients and for medical professionals.

THE FAMILY PERSPECTIVE

When a family brings a loved one to a hospital, their assumption is that they will receive the best care while admitted. That absolutely *should* be the case. But frustration and anger may occur when they notice their loved one is not doing well, especially if they feel that a lack of understanding of PD contributed to the poor outcome.

Unpredictable events can occur in the hospital, independent of how much the staff knows about PD. A sick patient can worsen in the hospital because that's unfortunately sometimes part of the disease process. Family members understand this and know that sometimes the length of stay will be long. What upsets them is when they see that the hospital isn't making an effort to improve the factors that can help the patient recover more quickly and leave the hospital better off. If those things can be done, they should be. If they're not, we certainly understand the family's frustration.

This is where family members need to be vocal and speak up on behalf of their loved one. If they feel that something isn't being done properly or hasn't been done well, they must say so. If family members feel that the patient isn't receiving the appropriate medicine or isn't getting it on time, they should tell the nurse, as well as the doctor who admitted the patient, and any other doctors involved with the patient's care.

Telling only one nurse doesn't ensure that the message gets through to the doctor or even to the other nurses. Family members and caregivers should speak with them and explain, firmly and calmly, that this is not how the patient is supposed to take his medicine, and then provide the appropriate instructions, including the timing and specific medications. If there are any questions, family members should put the hospital nurse and doctor in touch with the neurologist.

Sometimes the message still doesn't get heard. Family members who feel they're not getting through need to take action quickly to keep their loved one from going downhill. If, for example, a drug isn't on the formulary and the hospital staff is being difficult about it, family members may need to be very vocal about getting it or letting the patient take it from their home supply. Asking the patient's neurologist to intervene may be necessary.

Every hospital has patient advocates who are skilled at rallying the troops when there's an issue with care. They exist to help solve problems; caregivers and families should never hesitate to reach out to these people for help at any time. They go by different titles in different hospitals—patient advocates, patient representatives, care managers, ombudsmen, consumer advocates; every hospital has some form of patient advocacy, which can be helpful in such situations.

COGNITIVE IMPAIRMENT

All the problems a PD patient encounters in the hospital become more challenging if the patient is also cognitively impaired. The situation can be very frustrating for the family. Hospital staff have a tendency to treat cognitively impaired PD patients as if they have Alzheimer's disease and to not recognize that the impairment may have a different source and different characteristics.

People with PD can be cognitively impaired for many reasons. It might be due to their baseline problems, or to the inevitable progression of the disease, or because medication issues and the confusing hospital environment have tipped the patient into further impairment. Cognitive impairment is also a side effect of PD drugs.

When an inpatient is confused or showing other signs

of cognitive impairment, family and staff should think of the ABCs: appropriate medicine, best timing, and no contraindicated medications. Rule out medication problems; correct them if they exist.

Doctors, nurses, and other staff shouldn't assume that a confused patient is at their baseline. The confusion may be only temporary or drug-related. It is important to establish how this patient had been prior to the hospitalization. A hospital is fast-paced, and there may not be a lot of continuity of care—the staff may not have the time to get to know the patient before handing care off to the next shift. It's just easy to assume the patient has always been that way.

When a patient with PD seems confused or delirious, it's probably because of a medication issue. The first step is to check the meds and make sure all has been done correctly. If in doubt, nurses should consult caregivers and family members to confirm the correct drug, doses, and schedule. They also have to ensure that a medication has not been substituted and that a contraindicated medication has not been administered. If an adjustment is needed, it may be enough to get the patient from a state of confusion or delirium back to normal—back to their true baseline.

OBSTACLES TO CARE

Parkinson's disease medicine should be ordered in a customized fashion. Doctors and nurses should not rely on the EMR default dosing. When a medication should be taken five times a day, the usual default EMR dosing is 5:00 a.m., 9:00 a.m., 1:00 p.m., 5:00 p.m., and 9:00 p.m. In reality, that patient may take their medication at 6:00 a.m., 8:30 a.m., 11:00 a.m., 1:30 p.m., and 4:00 p.m., based on a schedule that they have worked out with their neurologist and that serves them best. While it is still five times daily, and their medication bottle will likely say 5x daily, this simple change in timing can significantly and negatively impact the patient in the hospital. The schedule should be customized to the patient's individual needs, and the drugs should be taken at whatever intervals work for them at home.

We have to reflect that schedule in the hospital setting, even if that means going through a few extra steps in the EMR to do it. People with Parkinson's are usually on a lot of medication at high doses. EMRs often trigger an error message that the dose is much higher than a normal dose. Someone admitting the patient, if they do not know the patient or know about PD, may decide to follow the EMR's recommendation for a lower dose, which is a potential disaster for the patient. Rather than blindly following an algorithm, doctors need to communicate with the patient and caregivers to determine exactly what meds the patient is on and order exactly that.

When such drug error warnings are presented by the EMR, they present an obstacle to providing the right medication for a patient. When the hospital pharmacy calls questioning the drug dosage, it again presents an obstacle to the care of the patient, as does receiving a call from the pharmacist saying a drug isn't available and suggesting a substitution. As providers, we have to be aware that PD patients may be on very high doses of medications. As long as we have confirmed the dose and the timing with the patient, the caregiver, or the patient's neurologist, we should insist on maintaining that same regimen while in the hospital.

These obstacles inhibit initiative and prevent the staff from providing excellent care. The system is designed to have checks and balances to avoid errors, but sometimes these safety measures aren't in the best interests of people with PD.

Particularly if a healthcare provider is relatively new to the hospital, overriding the EMR system may be difficult. And if the provider isn't familiar with Parkinson's, it adds to the dilemma. When they see that a patient is taking 10 times the EMR-recommended dose, they might decide that can't possibly be right and order whatever is recommended. They're overcautious because they don't want to harm the patient, but in fact, that's exactly what they're doing. If unsure, they should reach out to the family member or prescribing doctor. It's extra work, but it's the care we're supposed to provide for the patient. And it will save a lot of work later on, when the patient starts to go downhill because the doses are too low.

Be aware of the issues. Communicate with everyone involved, starting with the patient. There is a tendency to talk only to the caregiver, even when the patient is sitting right there and capable of answering. Ask the patient first and take the time to really listen to the answer, even if the patient has speech difficulties. Take the time to make sure communication is going both ways. The patient's masked expression doesn't mean lack of comprehension. Above all, adhere closely to the schedule, administer medications effectively, and avoid contraindicated medications.

LENGTH OF STAY AND HOSPITAL ECONOMICS

Studies show that people with PD end up having a hospital length of stay longer than those without PD. When we carry that number across the number of patients who are admitted per hospital, per town, per state, and nationally, the cost adds up to many millions of dollars. These extra costs could be largely avoided by better education about PD for doctors and hospital staff.

Hospitals are generally reimbursed a flat fee based on the diagnosis of the patient. What goes into that payment is a calculation of how many days that particular patient is expected to stay in the hospital. When patients stay longer than what is expected, in effect the hospital is penalized, because it doesn't get paid for the extra days. Lack of attention to medications can cause complications for patients who have PD and are in the hospital, and these then result in increases in length of stay for these patients. It's not surprising to see that poor medication management for PD patients is not only bad for the patients, but it's also bad for the hospital. In addition, if a patient is discharged from the hospital and is readmitted within a certain period, some health insurers penalize the hospital by not paying for the second hospitalization at all. These issues can also be avoided by paying close attention to medications, proper dosages, and proper timing and ensuring no contraindicated medications are administered when a patient is discharged, particularly when they are discharged to a rehab facility.

By giving the right medications on time every time, we can help the bottom line of the hospital by ensuring that Parkinson's patients leave on schedule and don't end up bouncing back because we didn't pay attention to their dosing and contraindicated medications. The additional advantage to the hospital of paying more attention is that patient bounce-back affects their public rankings and ratings. Reducing the bounce-back rate raises the ranking.

CHAPTER 8

Other Issues for Admitted Parkinson's Disease Patients

Admitted Parkinson's disease patients, whether for emergency treatment or elective surgery, have special needs that must always be considered.

THE PERIOPERATIVE PD PATIENT

In an ideal world, every PD patient would have an anesthesia consult before the surgery. In reality, a consult only happens when we're particularly worried about a patient who already has a major medical morbidity and needs elective surgery. We live in a world of limited resources, and a lot of what should be done simply can't be done. However, when someone who has more advanced Parkinson's needs surgery, a preoperative anesthetic consult makes sense. It will not only alert the anesthesiologist about special precautions for the patient, but it will also, we hope, avoid the risk of administering some postanesthesia medications that should not be given to a Parkinson's patient.

As discussed earlier, surgical patients should always get their PD meds before surgery and as soon after surgery as possible, even if they are NPO (nothing by mouth). This very clear pitfall is easy to avoid. Patients should take their medicines as usual up until the time of surgery, even if that's only minutes before. If the procedure lasts beyond the window for the patient's medication—it's a six-hour surgery but the drugs are usually taken every three hours, for example—then the drugs should be given as soon as the patient enters the recovery room. This might mean bending the rules a bit to give the patient their own medications. Even if they're incapable of swallowing at this point, crushing the tablet and putting it on the patient's tongue is often enough to get some of the drug into their system. Getting the patient back onto the usual dosing schedule as soon as possible after surgery is critical.

In our hospital, when a patient with PD comes in for elective surgery, an informational flyer about Parkinson's medications and contraindicated medications is attached to the chart. This flyer goes with them wherever they go through the hospital. Before the surgery, the anesthesiologist sees it in the operating room. After the surgery, it remains with the patient in the recovery room and beyond. It's another constant reminder we use, alerting all providers that this person has Parkinson's and needs to be taken care of correctly.

DEEP BRAIN STIMULATORS

If the patient has a deep brain stimulator, they may or may not be able to have an MRI. To know for certain if an MRI is possible, contact the implant manufacturer. The patient should have that information on a wallet card. Instructions about what to do and whom to call will be on the card. If the patient doesn't have the card, contact the surgeon or the patient's neurologist, who can provide more information.

Here are the two FDA-approved manufacturers and their contact information:

Medtronic Neuromodulation Patient Services: 1-800-510-6735

Abbott Scientific Technical Support 1-800-727-7846, option 3

ANESTHESIA

If anesthesia is required, the anesthesiologist, surgeon, and PD doctor should consult to determine the best option. It's important to review the medications list to make sure the patient isn't on something that might interact with anesthesia. The anesthesia should be kept as light as possible to avoid making post-op confusion worse.

MOBILITY

Mobility in general is reduced for any patient in the hospital. The rooms are small, and we don't really encourage patients to leave their rooms because we need to know where they are and be able to take vitals, give meds, examine them, and so on. This reduction in mobility is bad for all patients, but it's particularly bad for Parkinson's patients. We encourage Parkinson's patients to be as mobile and active as possible. Physical activity is really key to prolonging independence as the disease progresses.

When PD patients come to the hospital, they feel the lack of mobility just from being there, and that's compounded by whatever illness or procedure they have. We have to be vigilant about keeping Parkinson's patients mobile and encouraging them to get out of bed.

Ensuring mobility can be a real problem in hospitals in general, particularly in hospitals where everything has to be ordered. If a doctor doesn't create a specific order to get the patient out of bed, the nurses won't take, or even allow, the patient to get up. This is very unfortunate. Most hospitals have moved past this, but some hospitals still have this system in place; by default, they assume patients require bed rest. The default should really be that patients are encouraged to get out of bed.

Parkinson's patients in the hospital should be ambulating. They should be moved to a chair at least twice a day and taken to the bathroom as needed. It's extraordinarily critical to be automatic about these things. The ordering doctor admitting a Parkinson's patient should routinely order physical therapy, order them to leave the bed as tolerated, order nurses to put them in a chair, and order ambulation twice a day. Parkinson's patients aren't more likely to get post-op infections than anyone else. We know, however, that immobility after surgery or immobility in general can cause problems and raise the risk of pneumonia, urinary tract infections, pressure ulcers, and surgical site infection. PD patients need to be mobilized after surgery as soon as possible. They should also be mobilized as much as possible during recovery. Because these patients have gait and balance problems, a physical therapy program should begin as soon as possible after the surgery and continue throughout the hospitalization.

Hospital staff should be extra alert to fall risk with Parkinson's patients. These patients are at high risk because of motor symptoms such a gait problems. If they don't get their medications on time, studies show that the chance of falling increases. This can become a catch-22 sort of problem. These patients need to be mobilized, but they're at greater risk of falling, so we're reluctant to mobilize them, but the less we mobilize them, the more likely they are to fall. The fall-risk bracelet makes the staff nervous, but keeping the patient in bed is the worst plan of action for them. Awareness really matters. We have to be aware of how important mobility is for these patients. We have to be aware of the importance of timing of medications. Only in this environment can we reconcile these two issues of being concerned about the fall—and indeed these patients can fall—and needing them to move. If we keep them in bed, it's a disaster.

In our hospital, we have developed a PD champion program. Hospitals employ this concept for a variety of disorders: someone on the staff, usually a nurse or a physician, is the resident expert on that condition. When a patient with the condition is admitted, the champion works to remind and educate the staff about important aspects of care. For our PD patients, the champion reeducates the staff and those involved about the importance of medication timing, contraindicated medications, and mobility.

FREEZING AND GAIT

When a patient's medications start to wear off, the patient can freeze up, often quite suddenly. This is when a fall can happen, so the nursing staff needs to be vigilant. Freezing is probably more upsetting for the staff than the patient—the patient is quite used to it.

For some reason, patients with more advanced Parkinson's often freeze in doorways. They're also more likely to be distracted or confused by busy floor patterns. Some tricks can be used to help a frozen patient get moving again. We're not sure why they work, but they're very helpful. Patients who freeze can still step over a line on the floor in front of them and start moving again. In fact, some walkers have a laser pointer attached to them. When a patient freezes, they hit the laser button, a line appears on the floor in front of them, and they can walk over it. At home, many patients put tape on the floor around doorways to provide the line and make it easier to move around the house. If there's no laser pointer, someone can put their foot right in front of the patient's foot to form a line. The patient can step over it and continue walking.

Music can also help with mobilization. When a patient listens to music on a portable device, walking is improved. The beat of the music may stimulate the brain. People with PD can be extremely disabled but still perform like everyone else in some specific tasks. They can dance without anyone realizing they have Parkinson's, but when they stop dancing, their gait immediately reveals they have Parkinson's. Some people can still play sports. When the actor Michael J. Fox plays ice hockey, he's completely fine, but as soon as he stops, his Parkinson's symptoms return.

In a hospital setting, if a patient is freezing more than

usual, there's a very good chance that it's a medication issue. Double check the medication. It's also possible that they're just freezing, perhaps from the stress of being in the hospital.

SWALLOWING ISSUES

Most patients with advanced Parkinson's have some degree of dysphagia. Some of these patients even have chronic aspiration, because the swallow apparatus that protects the lungs from inhaling food and liquids isn't working properly. People with swallowing issues must prevent aspiration, as it can cause severe pneumonia. A speech therapist can help with swallow training. When hospitals encounter patients with swallowing problems or chronic aspiration, however, the automatic response isn't to bring in the swallow specialist. It's to make the patient NPO. As we've discussed, this can become a disaster for Parkinson's patients if NPO means they don't get their medication, and their nutritional status goes down. The hospital has valid legal concerns about patients aspirating, but NPO should be applied on a case-by-case basis and should be avoided wherever possible. Alternatives should be tried, such as thickening agents and swallow training.

FAMILY FRUSTRATIONS

Working out the ideal medications program for a PD

patient is a time-consuming, lengthy, trial-and-error process. Designing a regimen of medication and mobilization is a painstaking procedure that needs a lot of input from the patient and the family. It's worth the trouble because it keeps the patient as mobile and independent as possible for as long as possible.

Imagine the frustration the patient and family feel when a hospitalization destroys the work of weeks in just a few days and leaves the patient in much worse condition. Three days of hospitalization could set the patient back three months. That's what happens when a patient doesn't receive their medications on time and isn't mobilized properly.

Of course the family and patient are frustrated. They've put in weeks and weeks of hard work, making minor adjustments, ensuring the medicine is taken exactly on time, making sure the patient sticks to a regimented walking and exercise schedule. Now they see the patient unable to move, and it's heartbreaking.

We always need to be aware of the effort it took to keep that advanced-stage Parkinson's patient at least semi-independent and out of the nursing home. The family has worked hard to prevent that, only to see the hospital staff make mistakes that force the patient to become dependent and in a nursing home.

Anyone who has taken care of a chronically ill patient knows the amount of both emotional and physical work taking care of someone requires. It's exhausting. To feel that your months of effort to keep that patient chugging along are lost in the course of a few days is beyond frustrating. Be patient with family members who may be angry and frustrated about the care their loved one has received. In the end, both healthcare providers and family members want what is best for the patient, and with communication and understanding, these obstacles can often be removed.

Conclusion

The care of hospitalized people with Parkinson's disease can be greatly improved through education. When everyone in the hospital appreciates the importance of providing medications on time, every time, they have taken a major step toward providing excellent care for this population. When everyone in the hospital understands about contraindicated medications and is aware of how fragile patients with advanced PD are, the care improves even more.

When we look back at the cases of Gloria and George, we can easily see how better education and communication could have led to better choices and happier endings. The downhill course for both patients was set early on by medication errors based on a poor understanding of PD. For Gloria, prolonged intubation could have been avoided if the emergency room team had had a better understanding of why she needed her PD medication so urgently—and if the team had been better able to get it to her. For George, missed doses before and right after his surgery could have been avoided if everyone, starting with the surgeon, had had a better understanding of the importance of timely dosing no matter what. Had he received his drugs on schedule, he could easily have been ambulated early on and sent home sooner with a functional new knee.

Beyond education, communication with patients, caregivers, and family members is key. Good communication leads to good outcomes. Multidisciplinary teams are the best approach to comprehensive care for people with PD. Within the team, good communication helps the patient and family with preventative measures that can keep the patient independent longer and out of the hospital as much as possible. When a hospital stay is needed, good communication helps avoid medication errors and complications that can lead to poor outcomes and set patients back.

Education and communication make the difference when people with PD need to be in the hospital. We hope that they will make a difference at your hospital and lead to good outcomes, good patient satisfaction, and a more enjoyable workplace.

We are always interested in sharing ideas about how best to treat people with PD. Please talk to us at 201-342-2550.

www.northjerseybrainspine.com

PARKINSON'S FOUNDATION

www.parkinson.org
helpline@parkinson.org
1-800-473-4636 (4PD-INFO)

MICHAEL J. FOX FOUNDATION

www.michaeljfox.org
1-800-708-7644

AMERICAN PARKINSON'S DISEASE ASSOCIATION

www.apdaparkinson.org
apda@apdaparkinson.org
1-800-223-2732

Further Reading and References

Aminoff MJ, Christine CW, Friedman JH, et al. Management of the hospitalized patient with Parkinson's disease: current state of the field and need for guidelines. *Parkinsonism Relat Disord.* 2011;17(3):139-145.

Anderson LC, Fagerlund K. The perioperative experience of patients with Parkinson's disease: a qualitative study. *AJN.* 2013;113(2):26-32.

Braak H, Tredici KD, Rüb U, de Vos RA, Jansen Steur EN, Braak E. Staging of brain pathology related to sporadic Parkinson's disease. *Neurobiol Aging.* 2003;24(2):197-211. doi: 10.1016/s0197-4580(02)00065-9.

Brennan KA, Genever RW. Managing Parkinson's disease during surgery. *BMJ.* 2010;341:990-993.

Buetow S, Henshaw J, Bryant L, O'Sullivan D. Medication timing errors for Parkinson's disease: perspectives held by caregivers and people with Parkinson's in New Zealand. *Parkinsons Dis.* 2010;2010. doi: 10.4061/2010/432983.

Chenoweth L, Sheriff J, McAnally L, Tait F. Impact of the Parkinson's disease medication protocol program on nurses' knowledge and management of Parkinson's disease medicines in acute and aged care settings. *Nurse Educ Today.* 2013;33(5):458-464.

Derry CP, Shah KJ, Caie L, Counsell CE. Medication management in people with Parkinson's disease during surgical admissions. *Postgrad Med J.* 2010;86(1016):334-337.

Fagerlund K, Anderson, LC, Gurvich O. Perioperative medication withholding in patients with Parkinson's disease: a retrospective electronic health records review. *Am J Nurs*. 2013;113(1):26-35.

Fahn, S, Parkinson Study Group, et al. Levodopa and the progression of Parkinson's disease. *N Engl J Med*. 2004 Dec 9;351(24):2498-508.

Gerlach OHH, Broen MPG, van Domburg PHMF, Vermeij, AJ, Weber WEJ. Deterioration of Parkinson's disease during hospitalization: survey of 684 patients. *BMC Neurology*. 2012;12:13.

Grosset KA, Grosset DG. Effect of educational intervention on medication timing in Parkinson's disease: a randomized controlled trial. *BMC Neurol*. 2007;7:20.

Hely MA, Reid WG, Adena MA, Halliday GM, Morris JG. The Sydney multicenter study of Parkinson's disease: the inevitability of dementia at 20 years. *Mov Disord*. 2008 Apr 30;23(6):837-44. doi: 10.1002/mds.21956.

Hou JG, Wu LJ, Moore S, et al. Assessment of appropriate medication administration for hospitalized patients with Parkinson's disease. *Parkinsonism Relat Disord*. 2012;18(4):377-381. doi: 10.1016/j.parkreldis.2011.12.007.

Lertxundi U, Isla A, Solinís MÁ, et al. Medication errors in Parkinson's disease inpatients in the Basque Country. *Parkinsonism Relat Disord*. 2017;36:57-62. doi: 10.1016/j.parkreldis.2016.12.028.

Martinez-Ramirez D, Giuigni JC, Little CS, et al. Missing dosages and neuroleptic usage may prolong length of stay in hospitalized Parkinson's disease patients. *PLoS One*.2015;10(4):e0124356.

Parkinson's Foundation. *Parkinson's Toolkit: Clinical Best Practices*. Miami, FL: Clinical Resources; 2014.

Rezai AR, Machado AG, Deogaonkar M, Azmi H, Kubu C, Boulis N. Surgery for movement disorders. *Neurosurgery*.2008;62(2):SHC-809-SHC-839.

Smyth, J. *The NEWT Guidelines for Administration of Medication to Patients with Enteral Feeding Tubes or Swallowing Difficulties*. 5th Ed. Wrexham, Wales: North East Wales NHS Trust; 2006.

About the Authors

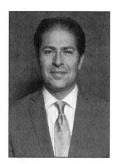

HOOMAN AZMI, MD, FAANS is director of the Division of Functional and Restorative Neurosurgery at Hackensack University Medical Center in New Jersey. He has authored numerous articles on the topic of Parkinson's disease and has lectured extensively on this subject. Dr. Azmi has spent the last 10 years developing innovative protocols and programs to improve the care of patients with Parkinson's disease, especially when they have been admitted to the hospital.

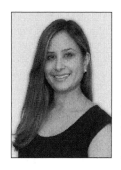

FIONA GUPTA, MD is a board-certified neurologist and fellowship-trained movement disorders specialist. She is director of the Movement Disorders Outreach Program at Mount Sinai Health Systems and an assistant professor of neurology.

Made in the USA
Middletown, DE
30 November 2018